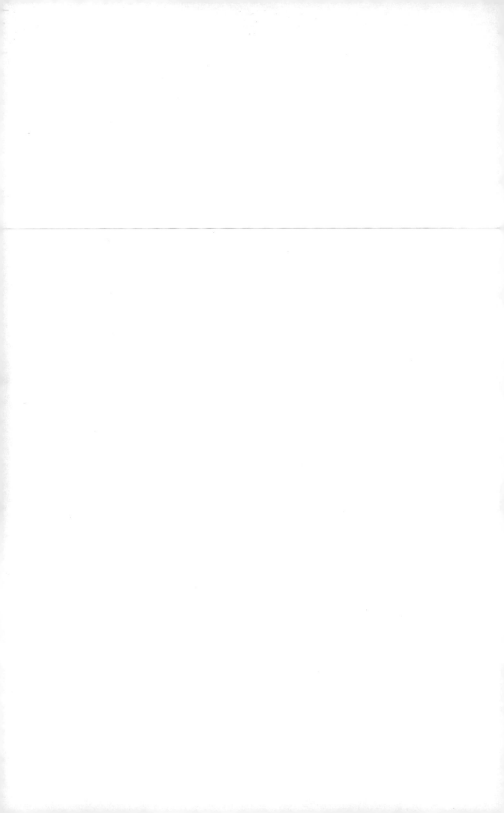

CHANGING THE WAY WE DIE

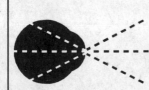

CHANGING THE WAY WE DIE

COMPASSIONATE END-OF-LIFE CARE AND THE HOSPICE MOVEMENT

FRAN SMITH AND SHEILA HIMMEL

Foreword by Joan Halifax, Ph.D.

THORNDIKE PRESS
A part of Gale, Cengage Learning

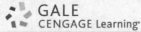

GALE
CENGAGE Learning·

Farmington Hills, Mich • San Francisco • New York • Waterville, Maine
Meriden, Conn • Mason, Ohio • Chicago

S

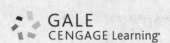

LIBRARY OF CONGRESS CATALOGING-IN-PUBLICATION DATA

Smith, Fran (Journalist), author.
  Changing the way we die : compassionate end-of-life care and the
hospice movement / by Fran Smith and Sheila Himmel ; foreword by Joan
Halifax, Ph.D. — Large print edition.
    pages cm — (Thorndike Press large print health, home & learning)
  Reprint of: Street Berkeley, California : Viva Editions, 2013.
  Includes bibliographical references.
  ISBN-13: 978-1-4104-6803-1 (hardcover)
  ISBN-10: 1-4104-6803-8 (hardcover)
  1. Hospice care—United States. 2. Terminal care—United States. 3. Death.
4. Compassion. I. Himmel, Sheila, author. II. Title.
  R726.8.S65 2014
  616.02'9—dc23   2013047810

Published in 2014 by arrangement with Viva Editions, an imprint of
Cleis Press Inc.

Printed in the United States of America
1 2 3 4 5 6 7 18 17 16 15 14

For our parents,

Dorothy and Carl Smith
Elaine and David Highiet

TABLE OF CONTENTS

FOREWORD

This beautiful book opens the lid on one of the most important treasures in our lives — how we can change the way we die. *Changing the Way We Die* reminds us that we often can choose to enter the embrace of hospice, with its deep roots in the heart of compassionate care.

Hospice in the United States has been a movement as well as a practice. Dedicated, sensitive professionals and volunteers bring love and care to those who are facing death, in their homes, hospital rooms, and freestanding hospices.

The words of patients and hospice people that fill this book reflect great wisdom and self-honesty. They are a testament to the vision of Dr. Cicely Saunders, the founder of the first modern hospice, St. Christopher's, in England.

I was honored in 1972 to spend time in St. Christopher's with Dr. Saunders. Hospice was just beginning to find a footing in the States. It is now a global practice and has given death the dignity it deserves.

I am grateful to the authors of this inspiring book.

Joan Halifax, Ph.D.
Upaya Zen Center
Santa Fe, New Mexico

INTRODUCTION

Nobody wants to die badly. Hospice care offers the best hope for dying well and living fully until we do. It should be routine, like surgery for appendicitis or antibiotics for a bacterial infection. But it is not, because hospice occupies a strange, uneasy place in the health care system, in the popular imagination, and in a famously youth-obsessed society that does not like to think about mortality.

We wrote this book to lift hospice out of the shadows. We set out to explore how its compassionate, holistic approach is changing the way Americans die and how its principles can be integrated into health care broadly, to improve care for everyone. We discovered that hospice is much more than a way to relieve the discomforts of dying. It is a way to live.

Hospice use is soaring, yet most people come too late to get the full benefits. Most

Americans want to die at home, not in hospitals, hooked up to machines. And with hospice help, more people are dying at home, but often only after tumultuous hospital stays and intensive, sometimes painful, ultimately futile last-ditch measures — surgery, a ventilator, a feeding tube, one more dose of chemo.

Hospice is the most successful segment of the health care system, in family satisfaction and cost effectiveness, yet it is widely feared and misunderstood. Many people think hospice is a place, and not a place you'd ever want to go. A friend — smart, worldly, accomplished — told us that she thought hospice was like a "parking garage where you're waiting to die." Hospice is not a place but a philosophy about living, dying, and dignity, and a set of practices to ease suffering. It does not mean giving up. Against all expectations, hospice care can open up time and emotional space for hope and healing.

Just as the age tsunami hits America and the need for end-of-life care grows, increasing commercialization by big business threatens hospice as we know it. For-profit hospices account for all the growth in the field over the past decade, and, as we show in the book, this shift raises troubling questions.

Meanwhile, 8,000 people turn sixty-five every day, and will for the next sixteen years. We need great hospice care more than ever.

In our research, we sat at the bedsides of patients, talked with families, followed around doctors and nurses, and interviewed some of the founders of the hospice movement in America. Among the many truths we learned, we both found this to be the most resonant:

When people acknowledge that dying is not "if" but "when," the essential question is: What do you want to do with the rest of your life?

About 1.5 million Americans a year die in hospice care — 44 percent of all deaths. A $14 billion industry serves the growing demand. Hospices seem to be everywhere — in nursing homes, hospitals, and prisons. You can even get hospice for your pet when the time comes. In some communities, competition for dying patients drives hospices to advertise on AM radio, like car-donation hustlers and the makers of anti-wrinkle creams. Shares of hospice companies trade on Wall Street.

We've come a long way since the early days, just forty years ago, when a handful of crusaders started the hospice movement. They met with derision and hostility. Was hospice a New Age indulgence? A quasi-religious practice? A rejection of wondrous medical advances? Many skeptics believed the movement would fade, certain that no red-blooded American would just go home and die rather than fight like hell, try every technological marvel out there, until that final breath.

The skeptics were wrong about the movement, but right about something deeper. Call it denial, blind optimism, or faith in the curative power of medical science — there is a collective resistance to accepting death as inevitable and to seriously planning for it. When we started telling people about this project, the less they knew about hospice the more warily they reacted. "Why hospice?" some friends asked, stiffening or subtly leaning away, as if we had a contagious disease. "Isn't it depressing?" Nurses and doctors who work in hospice get used to these questions and to the implication: that the experiences of the dying are far removed from the concerns of the living.

But people who had hospice support while caring for a dying loved one and those who wished they had, after watching someone die without it, eagerly shared their stories.

Strangers did too. The first time we met our book agent, in a busy café near Manhattan's Union Square, we talked about hospice for nearly an hour. As we stood to leave, a woman alone at the next table came over, admitted to eavesdropping, and told us about the wonderful hospice care her late husband had received. Again and again people said they wished they'd known about hospice sooner.

Our own losses planted the seeds for the book. Our fathers died around the same time, Fran's in a hospital, Sheila's in hospice care. We talked about what happened and how we felt about it, as friends do. It is always sad when a life winds down, but we realized that it does not have to be awful. With Fran's dad it was.

FRAN: My mother was alone by his side at the Veterans Administration Hospital in Brooklyn. As his breathing turned shallow and labored, she stroked his hand and whispered, "It's OK. You can rest now. I'll be fine. Go to sleep." Then, as if on cue, he did. She told me this when I arrived about forty minutes later. It was a cold January morning.

"Where were you?" she asked me. Simple question or accusation?

15

Before I could answer, she broke down in sobs.

I had taken the night shift. We did not call it that, but in those shapeless days, as my father lay there with pneumonia, my mother, my brother, and I fell into a pattern of taking turns, spelling each other: I'll stay, you eat, I'm not hungry, get some sleep. We knew the end was imminent. It was his second hospitalization for pneumonia in a month. This time we decided against antibiotics. My father had checked off this option on the advance directive that he had signed years earlier — and that we'd looked at, for the first time, just days before. But what was supposed to happen next? The directive did not hint at what my ninety-year-old father would have wanted as the clock ran down. Should my brother and I keep vigil? Did he want his wife of fifty-seven years to witness his death by herself? Did she?

Nobody on the hospital staff brought up such questions, and we did not think to raise them. Nobody mentioned hospice, and we did not ask for it. Instead: You eat, I'll stay, should I pick up milk on the way home?

My father had vanished long before he died, slipping away into dementia and almost complete physical incapacity. It started just before my husband and I had

16

our daughter. At her first birthday party, she and my father both knocked around with their walkers. He joked about it, we all did, as if he, like the baby, would soon outgrow the contraption and run free. Over time, I realized they were like two arms of an X, intersecting at a single point as she developed and he declined. He shed the walker not long after she did, because he needed a wheelchair. A year or so later, when I no longer had to buy diapers, my mother began to order them in bulk. By the time my daughter learned to write her name, he did not remember anyone's.

Sitting beside him that last night, I silently begged him to talk to me. Families often hope for a miracle, and this was mine. "Hey Daddy, it's me," I said, more than once. And then, partly to fill the silence, "I love you."

Late at night a nurse came, all brisk efficiency. After she left, I slid onto the bed's edge, and his eyes flew open and met mine. His gaze seemed clear, focused. "Hey Daddy," I said. "I'm so happy to see you."

I wanted to believe he recognized me. More likely it was I who recognized him, able at last to see my father inside the shell he had become.

"Look at that!" said the nurse, who had

come back. "He's smiling at you."

After he fell asleep, I drove back to my mother's apartment to nap and shower. When I woke up, she had already left for the hospital. I scrambled to get ready and join her, but on the way I decided to run an errand. Even the most astute hospice professional cannot predict the moment of death, but I have wondered whether I would have been at my father's bedside that morning if our family had known more about what to expect.

I have wondered even more what his life in the lead-up would have looked like had hospice been involved, or any professional with the will and skill to talk frankly about dying and the decisions ahead. He died peacefully, but after years of hell for everyone, him especially. He had been treated for infections and other ailments in his last years. In hindsight, we could have said no to antibiotics much earlier. I know he would not have wanted to live utterly helplessly, as he did. But nobody asked if we wanted to consider an alternative, and the possibility never crossed our minds.

SHEILA: My father turned toward the daylight the moment before he died, as if following a movie script. The dutiful elder son, he believed in doing things the right way. On a sunny Easter morning, Mom, my sister, and I crunched around his diminished body in the nursing home bed. Mom and Nancy each held a hand while I rubbed his bony shoulder. We cried, told him we loved him, and said we'd be OK; he could go. He hadn't been conscious in many days, hadn't eaten in a week. His feet were cold and blue, his skin papery gray. His breaths got raspier and more startling — the proverbial rattle — and further apart. Then, he wasn't there anymore. We waited for another breath, but his spirit had flown away and left its lifeless casing, like a husk. It was so peaceful. There had been four of us in the room, and now there were three.

All the elements of active dying we knew to be normal because the hospice nurse had told us. For four and a half months, we had the hospice nurses, social worker, aides, and a 24-hour hotline to ask about what might happen next. He died a month after turning eighty-three, officially from heart failure. The California death certificate requires one immediate cause of death.

Three years earlier, dementia had descended, and instability on his feet. He stayed in bed and was uninterested when people came to visit. Mom hired a companion, who helped a lot until Dad became incontinent. The man didn't change diapers.

As months went by, he fell, setting off alarms and hospitalizations, each time coming back weaker, like a broken prizefighter on the way down. Still, he clung to a tradition he had followed in business and personal matters — weighing the facts, making a plan, doing things right. For a while, being in a nursing home was the right choice. He became his friendly self again, and got up for meals and occupational therapy. Until he didn't. The nursing home staff suggested it might be time to consult hospice.

Again, life improved temporarily. Medications were simplified, side effects eliminated, including dizziness that may have been caused by the blood pressure medication he'd been taking for years. There would be no more badgering him to go to OT, no more ambulances. It was as if a shroud of anxiety had lifted because we could ask someone what was OK, what to do or say that might help him or us. We could just sit there with him, talking, holding his hand. Thanks to the hospice nurses, we knew he didn't have to do anything.

As they told us he would, Dad grew weaker and more confused until the intermittent responsive days dwindled to a stop.

In the last weeks, he wasn't in pain, but it was as if he was visiting elsewhere while his body stayed in bed.

On a Friday in April, the hospice nurse told Mom he would likely die in the next day or so. My sister, Nancy, and her family again flew in from Seattle.

Saturday afternoon we gathered in Dad's room, with cards, photos, and kids' art on the walls, and started talking about funeral arrangements. "Just so you know, hearing is the last sense to go," the nurse said, not unkindly. We had to laugh, because Dad wouldn't have minded: We were making plans so that things would be done right.

The Long Road to the End

Our own experiences got us thinking about the difference that hospice can make, but they do not make us experts. Our training and instincts as journalists are to make sense of complicated situations by documenting other people's experiences. That's why we collected so many stories from people on both the receiving and the giving ends of hospice care. With their consent, we use only real names — no composites or invented details to protect anonymity. Hospice can emerge from the shadows only if we all see how it works for people living

21

lives as real, as rich, and as flawed as anyone else's.

Death comes differently today than at any other time in history. Most of us are not likely to have the swift, sudden death of a virulent infection, the leading cause of death until the twentieth century. We probably will not die in an instant of a heart attack (or in a plane crash, a terrorist attack, or any of the headline-making catastrophes we worry about). Sanitation and modern medicine have transformed dying from a quick, unhappy event that takes loved ones by surprise into a gradual process.

We have time to anticipate the end. Families have time to prepare. That may sound like a curse. *Changing the Way We Die* shows that hospice can make it a gift.

Part One, The Choice, explains what hospice is all about. Why do people suffer? Can hospice care really bring relief? How? Why don't more people seek such help? We trace these questions back to the founding of hospice, when high ideals created a revolutionary way of caring for the dying only to collide with economic and political realities.

Part Two, The Patients, focuses on the decisions that hospice has allowed some people to make — and the outcomes of those decisions. What prompts people to turn to hospice? How do they know the time is right? What is their experience? Do their loved ones have regrets? We tell very different stories — from a young father who loved the care he received in hospice only to get transferred out, to a ninety-one-year-old woman whose fifteen months on hospice got her walking again, visiting favorite places, and meeting her first great-grandchild. We profile a man who fasted to death rather than suffer a slow, torturous decline, and a man who endured years of brutal cancer treatments to buy every bit of extra time.

Part Three, The Survivors, looks at one of the most underappreciated aspects of hospice care: the help it gives families not only while a loved one is dying, but also afterward. How do survivors look back on the time in hospice? How does hospice help them get on with their lives? What have they learned about dying, living, and the choices we all will face?

Part Four, The Providers, goes inside the rapidly changing hospice universe. How does hospice help people find meaning or face death if they don't believe in God or an afterlife? Why do some doctors choose to work with patients they cannot cure? And what about patients who can be cured — shouldn't modern medicine work to ease their suffering too? How did Wall Street discover hospice and alter hospice? Will hospice survive?

Although making the choices that hospice affords is never easy, perhaps it's easier when a loved one is old and failing, like our fathers. We begin with a man named Rusty Hammer, who faced the choices in the prime of life.

■ ■ ■ ■

PART ONE:
THE CHOICE

■ ■ ■ ■

CHAPTER ONE:
WHAT DO YOU WANT TO DO WITH THE REST OF YOUR LIFE?

"Oh no, he's giving up.
He's just going to die."

All along, doctors differed on Rusty Hammer's prognosis. One told his wife, Pamela, "If he lasts five years, he'll be lucky." Another kept reassuring Rusty, "You never know. You're doing fine. Just get more rest."

He did last five years, but Pamela will always wonder whether the treatment was worth the torment.

Rusty was diagnosed with acute myelogenous leukemia, a rare and aggressive blood cancer. By the time he died, on Monday, January 28, 2008, he had taken more than 250 medications, received more than 350 blood transfusions, had a stem cell transplant, and spent nearly 600 nights in six different hospitals. He developed severe diabetes and osteoporosis, heart and lung failure. He needed an oxygen tank for breathing and a shunt in his brain to relieve the pain. Visiting the doctor took all day, with the wheelchair, the drive, managing a hospital bed on the other end. It left them both exhausted, and hopeless that their family's suffering would ever end.

But hospice care brought them comfort and calm. In the last six months of his life, Rusty enjoyed the company of family and friends. He explored his religious heritage. He wrote a book, and in a strange way he also became the author of his own experience — a person again, not a medical record number or an object to be handed from one specialist to another for yet another debilitating treatment. The hospice team listened to him. Pamela found herself becoming a better listener too.

This was not how Rusty thought of hospice when a friend first suggested it. He did not imagine an opportunity to reclaim his life, let alone do something new or grow. He thought of hospice as a place you go to die, and he was appalled.

The Best Medicine
Rusty's fear is common, as is the desire not to die in a hospital. By better than two to one, Americans consistently say they want to die at home, without pain, among the

people they love. As they tell pollsters: no breathing tube down the throat, electrodes plastered to the chest, IV lines snaking from arms. In a March 2011 poll of 1,000 adults by the Regence Foundation and *National Journal,* 71 percent said it is more important to improve the quality of life of a seriously ill patient than to extend life through every medical intervention conceivable.

Hospice delivers on these wishes. It is the best medicine for dying patients and their families when quality of life, however a person defines that, is the goal. Nothing else in health care matches it for breadth of services or compassion. If you are sixty-five or over, Medicare pays. Medicaid does too, and many private insurance plans.

In medical literature, where just about every treatment, innovation, and guideline seem to stir controversy and confuse rather than clarify the best choices, there is no dispute about the benefits of hospice. And, in an economy where every expense is on the table, the cost-effectiveness of hospice cannot be ignored.

The rapid growth of hospice speaks to its appeal and to the depth of our collective desire for a better way of dying. The first hospice in the United States, in New Haven, Connecticut, began caring for patients in

1974. Four years later, fifty-nine hospice programs served patients (though only a handful in most cases). The 1981 directory of the fledgling National Hospice Organization listed 464 hospices in operation and 353 trying to get off the ground. Just about all these groups ran on the sweat and dreams of volunteer nurses, clergy, doctors, and social workers. Today there are more than 5,000 programs. A cadre of end-of-life experts is developing ever more refined techniques to control pain and other symptoms. Medical schools do a better job of teaching students about the once unmentionable subject of dying. Fellowship programs train hundreds of young physicians a year in hospice care and palliative medicine.

Yet, even as hospice gains ground, the use of aggressive last-gasp medical interventions is increasing. From 2000 to 2009, hospice use among Medicare patients nearly doubled, to 42 percent. But more patients enrolled in hospice only after aggressive treatment in intensive care units in the final weeks and months of their lives. Nearly one in six patients was moved from one setting to another in the last three days — from home to a hospital, for instance, or from the hospital back to the nursing home. For too many patients, hospice was just another quick stop in a chaotic journey through a fragmented health care system.

The fear of death and the resistance of the medical profession prevent many of us from embracing the opportunities hospice affords to live the end of our lives in a way we find meaningful and to have the kind of death we say we want. Medicare and many insurance plans cover hospice care for people with a life expectancy of six months, and if you happen to live longer, you can remain on hospice or leave until your condition worsens. But the median length of service is just nineteen days. Thirty-six percent of hospice patients die within a week of enrollment. Rabbi Mychal Springer, director of the Center for Pastoral Education at the Jewish Theological Seminary in New York, trains seminary students of diverse faiths to provide pastoral care in hospices, and she says her students are always shocked to discover that, by the time they are called in, many patients can no longer communicate or seem to register their presence.

Waiting until the very end to choose hospice, clinging to the sliver of hope that the next new drug or procedure will bring the miracle, diminishes the possibility of dying well. It robs patients of the time and energy to hug a loved one goodbye or to sit in the sunshine of the garden or to stroke the soft fur of a beloved pet or to tie up loose ends financially, emotionally, and spiritually. "If you sign up for hospice and you have twenty-four to forty-eight hours left to live, you're not up for very much," Springer said, perhaps stating the obvious. "It's such a waste."

The Hammers would take a different path.

"All I Wanted to Do Was Go Home for Good"

Rusty Hammer thought hospice meant giving up, and he was not a quitter. All his life, he took action, blazed trails. At the age of eighteen, he had been voted onto the city council in Campbell, California, becoming the youngest elected official in United States history. Now Campbell is just another dot on the map of Silicon Valley, but back then it was a cannery town surrounded by orchards. His election was the biggest thing to happen there since the invention of fruit cocktail, to which Campbell laid a claim. While on the council, Rusty attended the University of Santa Clara full time and worked at Steve's Pharmacy in downtown Campbell. In 1975, he became the nation's youngest mayor ever elected, an accomplishment covered by such wide-ranging news outlets as *Seventeen* and the *London Times*. The *National Enquirer* headlined the story, "Youngest Mayor is Only 22." For once, the tabloid downplayed the story; Hammer was twenty-one.

As mayor, Rusty worked with a vocal advocate for disabled access, a woman who had been paralyzed by polio. She liked the earnest young man presiding at long, contentious meetings. She went home and told her daughter, Pamela, "Oh, I've met this wonderful man." Nine months later, Rusty and Pamela were married.

Pamela gave birth to twins and Rusty went on to a career as a corporate and nonprofit executive. As years went by, they moved to Florida, to Sacramento, and then to Los Angeles, where he ran the Chamber of Commerce. When the twins, Gerald and Jennifer, were about to graduate from college and Rusty was turning fifty, his back started hurting. The Hammers and their doctors thought it was from an auto accident, but the pain persisted and a PET scan lit up a mass of tumors. The orthopedic surgeon who had ordered the scan said, "I think we have bigger issues than your back."

Rusty had a surgical biopsy. Diagnosed with acute myelogenous leukemia, with a

20 percent chance of living five years, he was hospitalized in preparation for a bone marrow transplant. After two weeks of high-dose chemotherapy to clear up the cancer as much as possible, his white blood cell count dropped dangerously low and his stomach became infected. Then he developed symptoms of congestive heart failure. The bone marrow transplant was postponed, and it was six weeks before he was allowed to go home, for five days.

"All I wanted to do was go home for good," he later wrote. "I kept going back to the hospital over and over again."

Instead of the bone marrow transplant, Rusty's doctor decided to do a less painful stem cell transplant. He was hospitalized for four months. Then came a cascade of complications, from diabetes induced by the steroids he was taking, to pneumonia, to a staph infection from a catheter.

When he was strong enough, the Hammers moved back to Silicon Valley to be closer to friends and family. Two or three times a week, Pamela got Rusty dressed and into the car for the half-hour drive to oncology appointments at Stanford Hospital. There they had to find a room supplied with oxygen equipment and wait, usually hours. Another season went by, and Pamela said,

"Rusty, what do you want to do?" He wanted to keep up the treatments. But Pamela was worn to the bone, he could see, and he felt responsible. "My illness was sapping Pamela's life," he later wrote.

Although Hospice of the Valley had been around almost thirty years — like Rusty, a local institution — he knew almost nothing about it. But, four and a half years after his diagnosis, he agreed to let a hospice worker come to the house — just to explain the services. He learned that Hospice of the Valley was not a building to house patients but a service that would come to him.

The social worker told him that, even in the final stages of a terminal illness, there are choices. Is there someone you need to mend fences with? Do you want to travel? See friends? Keep your family close? Is there work you want to finish? The young man distilled the essence for Rusty: "What do you want to do with the rest of your life?"

Some friends argued it was too soon. A relative, horrified, protested to Pamela, "Oh no, he's giving up. He's just going to die." But the social worker's list of choices took up residence in Rusty's mind. He wanted to spend time with Pamela, the twins, and his lifelong friends. He might even have time to write the book he'd been thinking about, to help other people deal with cancer. Rusty and Pamela had long talks: What *did* he want to do with the rest of his life?

That question gets to the heart of what hospice is all about. It is much more than physical comfort care. Relieving agony is of course important, and hospices have pioneered techniques to ease pain, breathing difficulties, agitation, and other distressing symptoms. These methods and the broader emphasis on relieving suffering are finally finding their way into hospitals, through palliative medicine services, to the enormous benefit of sick people who are not necessarily about to die.

But hospice services extend well beyond the medical. Hospice offers counseling, spiritual support, and help with practical issues, from filling out tax forms to arranging a visit from an estranged child. St. Christopher's Hospice in South East London, the first modern hospice and the lodestar for programs the world over, once allowed a circus owner determined to cheer up his dying father to bring a baby elephant to visit.

No hospice in America would go that far, but the ethic of expansive patient-driven care runs strong. Pets are often welcome to stop by inpatient hospices, and if a patient at home is too sick to care for a pet, many hospices will send a volunteer to help. It is not unusual to find hospices offering aromatherapy, massage, art therapy, life reviews, and music therapy. All these can forge almost magical connections with a patient who seems beyond reach. One spring day in an inpatient hospice unit in California, a harpist played in the room of a moaning, thrashing woman with cancer. The tone, pitch, and rhythm of the instrument matched the sounds of the patient, and soon she quieted and drifted off to sleep.

Underlying these practices is the concept of "total pain," a phrase coined by Cicely Saunders, the nurse-turned-social worker-turned-physician who founded St. Christopher's in 1967. Hospice care is built around the idea that anguish at the end of life does not stem only, or even primarily, from the physical ravages of disease. "Bodies don't suffer, people do," said Charles F. von Gunten, editor in chief of the *Journal of Palliative Medicine*. "The emotional component, the practical issues, the spiritual dimension — that's where the suffering is."

Another hallmark of hospice is its view of death not as failure but as an inevitable passage. If we face it honestly, we can prepare for it. If we prepare, we may find meaning, value, and deep human connection up to the very end.

Whether that sounds like common sense or wishful thinking, the perspective diverges sharply from the medical model and its almost exclusive focus on the mechanistic causes and treatment of illness. In a fundamental way, the hospice mission of helping people to die well runs counter to a medical system geared toward fighting death at all costs. On cancer wards, where hospices found their first patients, physicians initially viewed a specialty devoted to dying as a rebuke — "the antimatter of cancer therapy, the negative to its positive, an admission of failure to its rhetoric of success," Siddhartha Mukherjee writes in his history of cancer, *The Emperor of All Maladies*.

Physician attitudes have changed since the early days, but not enough. It is the unusual oncologist or heart specialist who presents hospice as the next step along the continuum of expert care, a program like any other in medicine, staffed by people highly trained to meet the particular, complex needs of patients at this phase of their lives. More commonly, hospice is offered up as the sad last resort, after doctors have tried everything and the patient has "failed" to respond. Sometimes hospice is not offered up at all.

When Rusty decided at last to sign up for care from Hospice of the Valley, his oncologist refused to sign off. Rusty was not going to die from his leukemia anytime soon, the doctor insisted. Normally respectful of authority and always polite, Pamela lost it. She fired off an angry email noting that they understood there was always one more thing to try, but time was limited. The doctor relented.

With hospice care, Rusty Hammer's symptoms were kept in check. Doctors, nurses, and medicines came to the house. The doctor stayed an hour each time — an hour!

Rusty set up shop in his recliner, with his computer, printer, phone, and side table, friends and family coming and going, talking about politics. His children, Gerald and Jennifer, visited often. The living room became a salon, and he presided over it with the same charm, humor, and intelligence that had gotten him elected to the city council so many years earlier.

In the living room, Rusty wrote about his cancer experience. He described chemotherapy, acknowledging, "We were most naïve about the side effects and risks of treatment at the various stages." He railed at hospital doctors who just prescribed painkillers and left the room, with never a palliative care consult or a referral to a pain specialist. "I am a living example that, in many cases, the treatment can be worse than the disease."

Students at a nearby high school were rehearsing *Wit,* a play about the final hours of an English professor dying from cancer. To better understand the play, they had done research about death and dying and read a Hospice of the Valley newsletter mentioning Rusty's forthcoming book. Students came to interview him. Rusty published *When Cancer Calls, Say Yes to Life,* and had a book party at the hospice offices. More than fifty people came, including the teen-agers involved with *Wit.*

Hours before Rusty died, he called to wish an old friend happy birthday. Another dear friend — the woman who had first suggested hospice — dropped by. The housekeeper was there that day, which usually gave Pamela a chance to run errands, but she had a feeling she should stay. Rusty worked the phones and his computer, and that night, in his recliner, his breathing changed. He told Pamela, "I love you," and nodded off.

For a long time afterward, even as she faced her future and joined a hospice-sponsored bereavement group, Pamela could not help but look back and think about how much suffering Rusty would have avoided had they considered hospice sooner.

Hospice should not be such a hard choice to make, but our health care system and even hospices themselves make it so. That's in large part because of the way hospice grew in America and because of the compromises it had to make as it matured, which brings us to the idealists who started it all.

CHAPTER TWO:
BIRTH OF A MOVEMENT

"Constant pain needs constant control."

The story begins with three women who did work nobody else wanted to do and said things many people did not want to hear. Each articulated ideals that lie at the core of the hospice approach and put them into action. Two of the women, Florence Wald and Cicely Saunders, met at Yale University in New Haven, Connecticut, in the spring of 1963.

Saunders had come to the Yale School of Medicine to talk about the hospice she was building in South East London. It was her first trip to the United States and the first time many Americans, even health care professionals, heard the word *hospice*. Only about forty people showed up for the lecture in Fitkin Amphitheater, a plunging semicircular hall that seated 150. Yet, as she stood by the lectern, elegant and just over six feet tall, she seemed to fill the room. In impeccable clipped speech that hinted at her posh English upbringing, Saunders claimed to achieve the unthinkable: keeping patients pain free, generally alert, and in some cases rather jolly, until just before they died.

She made it sound fairly easy to do. She said she freely administered oral narcotics, typically in a cocktail of heroin, honey, and whiskey, or brandy if a patient preferred. She also pushed care beyond the confines of medicine to address the spiritual, psychological, social, and practical needs of her patients and their families.

Even then, at the outset of a career that would inspire the creation of thousands of hospices around the world, earn her innumerable awards, and move Queen Elizabeth II to anoint her a Dame of the British Empire, the female version of a knight, Saunders knew how to work an audience. She flashed before-and-after photos of her patients on a screen behind her, to riveting effect. The slides showed people upon admission to her wards, disfigured and debilitated by cancer and its brutal treatments. Days, weeks, or months later, as death in her care drew near, there were those same patients smiling, serene, sometimes chatting with grandchildren dressed in their Sunday finest.

To anyone familiar with the agonizing downhill slope of dying patients in hospitals in the 1960s, the pictures looked like a movie in rewind — or a mistake. A few years after the Yale lecture, a young doctor named Doris Howell found herself operating the slide projector for Saunders during a similar talk in a Philadelphia church. Until that day, Howell knew nothing about hospice. The English doctor handed Howell before-and-after slides of fifty patients.

Saunders began her lecture and signaled for the first slide. Howell flicked it on screen, glanced up at what was supposed to be the "before" image and panicked.

"Oh my God, I've got the wrong slide," Howell thought.

"It was perfectly obvious I had just put in the slide of a patient lying on the gurney shrouded in a white sheet, and white as the sheet, obviously so near death, if not dead, and of course that was the patient at the time of death, or approaching death," Howell told an oral historian decades later. "So I shoved the slide carrier over as fast as I could, saying, 'I'm so sorry,' and Cicely is saying, 'No, no, no, no, no, no, go back, go back!' . . . And I'm saying, 'No, I have the wrong slide.' She's saying, 'You had the right slide.' " The man looked dead when he came to the hospice from a hospital.

But it was the paired slide, the later photo, that "just undid me, as it undid the rest of the audience," Howell said. The man was sitting up in bed with a dog by his side, a cocktail glass in his hand lifted as if in a toast to good health. As the audience gasped, marveling at his apparent turn-around, Saunders said he had died that night. "The audience was speechless," Howell recalled.

It wasn't only the pictures of course; the message also jolted audiences. Saunders was challenging a medical world that had focused for most of the past century on conquering diseases to at least consider the possibility that it had something to offer terminally ill people — a lot, in fact. She envisioned physicians teaming with nurses, social workers, chaplains, and even patients and families — this in a day when doctors reigned supreme, years before the words *multi-disciplinary, informed consent,* or, for that matter, *team* entered the lingo of health care. She also called for the continuous administration of narcotics, insisting, "Constant pain needed constant control." This too defied standard practice. Physicians often withheld morphine and other pain medicine until a patient's agony became intolerable or the screaming and thrashing became too awful for a family to witness, because everyone worried that patients, even dying ones, would become addicted.

Most astonishingly, Saunders believed that all decisions about care should be driven by the wishes of patients, not by the opinions of specialists or the convenience of nurses or the rules of hospitals, government health programs, or insurance companies. If a patient wanted to hear a violinist, confess to a priest, reconcile with an estranged sister, or keep that sister away, the hospice would arrange it. If a patient craved a steak or a spot of sherry, the hospice would serve it, and if a patient had no appetite, aides would whisk away the meal. No detail escaped Saunders's attention. She once received a fifty-dollar donation designated for "liquor" and promptly sent it to her brother Christopher, who was pitching in as her business manager. "Put this toward more wine," she instructed, "bearing in mind that patients will, on the whole, prefer red to white." She further recommended half-bottles. "I know they are tiresome to store but they might well be more acceptable to patients than the large ones."

Florence Wald missed Saunders's lecture

at Yale but heard about it from a nursing school colleague right after. Wald tracked down Saunders on campus and invited her to meet with the nursing faculty. Wald had never liked the way hospitals handled dying patients. She complained about "never-ending intensive treatment carried to the bitter end as patients suffered and became more helpless." It always pained her to see doctors evade the questions of terrified families: Is the treatment working? How long will it be? And it angered her that nurses often got caught in the middle, ignored or worse when they dared to nudge physicians to talk honestly with patients and families. "At best, nurses were rebuffed," Wald wrote. "At worst, they were barred from care."

Now here came Cicely Saunders, condemning these practices and creating a compassionate alternative. "Until then I had thought nurses were the only ones troubled by how a terminal illness was treated," Wald later wrote.

The day after Saunders spoke at the medical school, she met with Yale nurses. Florence Wald was hooked and soon made up her mind to start a program in Connecticut modeled on the British experiment. Wald's program would embrace the vision of patient and family in the foreground, with experts and medical intervention in the background. It would operate on the conviction that listening was an essential act of care. Maybe it would even adopt the alien title that Cicely Saunders used: *hospice.*

The word derived from the Latin *hospes,* meaning both guest and host, and it gave a mythic aura to the work of Cicely Saunders, Florence Wald, and other hospice pioneers in the 1960s and early 1970s. Saunders cultivated the mystique. In articles and speeches, she often harked back to the first places to be called hospices — Christian shelters that dotted the routes through Europe to the Holy Land from medieval days until around the seventeenth century. Run by monasteries, the shelters carried out the dictate of the Gospel of Matthew, Chapter 25: I was a stranger, and you welcomed me. Given the primitive state of medical care and the difficulty of travel, strangers often straggled in exhausted and sick. Those who recovered may have journeyed on, but many drew their final breath in the care of the monks.

These way stations for pilgrims provided a good foundation tale for a twentieth-century movement that had to battle for credibility. It was more appealing to conjure images of wayfarers and quests than to talk only about pain, death, and the failures of modern hospitals. Yet the original hospices differed fundamentally from the contemporary version. While they did not shun the dying, they did not exist to serve the dying, either. As science became a legitimate focus for inquiry in the 1800s and medical knowledge expanded, some of these shelters were converted into hospitals. No longer were monks confined to watching people die and praying for their souls. The impulse was to try to cure.

The hospices that directly influenced Cicely Saunders and the modern movement — the first British institutions to declare it their mission to serve the dying — sprang up in much grittier soil, in the Dickensian slums of England and Ireland. The Irish Sisters of Charity led the way (and gave new meaning to the h-word) with the founding of Our Lady's Hospice in Dublin in 1879. The Sisters wore the hospice mantle not because of any association with good care for the dying but because of the old connection to pilgrims. The Sisters saw death as a part of an eternal journey, a step toward salvation. They believed that, under their Catholic wing, even the poorest wretch from the sin-filled streets could be redeemed, but they also realized that pain and festering sores would distract from matters of the spirit. By offering salves, pain medicine, and other comfort measures, the Sisters held out a new kind of hope, for relief right here on earth.

Queen Victoria's Britain turned out to be fertile ground for pioneering work focused on the dying. Death was an obsession and, in elegant neighborhoods, quite the social affair. Victorian funerals were big, lavish, and ruled, as were most matters, by rigid rules of etiquette. In the mid-1800s, London's Regent Street was like a shopping mall for death, with four retail houses doing brisk sales in mourning attire and accoutrements — from the proper dress for morning versus evening to the correct hat to the suitable parasol. A nineteenth-century French writer marveled at the elaborate rituals. "The care the English take of all particulars of their burial would make one believe that they find more pleasure in dying than living," he observed.

He was referring to English people with money, of course, who expected to die at home, surrounded by loving relatives and attended by a doctor and a cleric. The deathbed scene looked bleaker in squalid neighborhoods — if the patient had a bed at all. Cancer was believed to be contagious, and people with visible tumors were often driven from their homes, to wind up in prison or the poorhouse. A newspaper appeal for funds for an early hospice in London described the plight of such unfortunates: "They died in conditions worse than the most savage of savages have ever yet had to face."

Those conditions led to the founding of St. Luke's Home for the Dying Poor in 1893 and St. Joseph's Hospice in 1905, two London institutions where Cicely Saunders would work early in her career and clarify her thinking about the needs of the terminally ill. Conditions were no better for destitute dying patients across the Atlantic. That drove a woman named Rose Hawthorne Lathrop to build two of the first facilities in the United States dedicated exclusively to the care of incurable cancer patients.

From Privilege to Purpose, and the Hawthorne Legacy

She was the youngest child of Nathaniel Hawthorne, author of *The Scarlet Letter* and other American classics, and Sophia Peabody Hawthorne, a descendant of a prominent early New England family. In the 1890s, when she was in her mid-forties, Rose Hawthorne Lathrop withdrew from her elite circle, became a devout Catholic, trained as a nurse, and opened Saint Rose's Free Home for Incurable Cancer in the slums of Manhattan's Lower East Side. With her pedigree and her prolific accounts of the suffering and the humanity of her patients, Lathrop drew considerable press coverage for her work. She also attracted big-name donors, among them author and family friend Samuel Clemens, better known as Mark Twain.

Decades before Cicely Saunders would outline the precepts of modern hospice care, Lathrop argued that everyone should have the right to die in dignity and peace. And she did everything possible to help patients die that way at Saint Rose's. The three-story brick townhouse must have seemed like Eden in the fetid neighborhood, with freshly painted shutters, white starched curtains, and easy chairs scattered about a garden. Lathrop and her volunteer helpers did all the nursing, because she insisted that care was an act of mercy, not a chore for hired hands. (She hired men to bathe and dress male patients.) Rooms were airy and bright, in accordance with her dictate that patients should be "as comfortable and happy as if their own people had kept them and put them into the very best bedroom." Although she used all the medications at her disposal and experimented with salves to relieve putrid sores, she considered a cheerful atmosphere to be "the best treatment of all." She indulged patients as much as her meager budget allowed. Her helpers sat on crates to eat meals because she could not afford enough chairs to go around, and patients got them first.

"The men will ask to venture outdoors with a pipe and a beer, an indescribable morale lift," she wrote. "The women sew and hold endless talking bees. . . . Many enjoy reading daily and weekly prints, writing letters and being soothed or frolicked by the phonograph's discourse of the most excellent music" — Enrico Caruso's tenor, Mischa Elman's violin, and the first choral hymns ever recorded, by the Sistine Chapel Choir.

This was a religious enterprise, like the British hospices of the same era. Lathrop forbade proselytizing and welcomed patients of all religions, or none, but she believed that she was preaching the gospel through nursing, and she rejoiced when someone came to the faith. Patients remained in her care as long as necessary. She accepted no payment for her services and relied on donations, as would the first American hospices, in the 1970s.

Lathrop called her band of helpers the Servants of Relief, but she was no docile handmaiden. She publicly condemned the institutional neglect of the dying poor and a medical system she saw as driven more by money than by human need.

"It is a mistake to erect a hospital which is a model of inventions, a triumph of arrangement, if the building is to be serviceable to the destitute," she wrote in *Christ's Poor,* a fiery monthly pamphlet she published for four years in the early 1900s. "Every penny accumulated should go to the benefit of the poor; not the greater share to the benefit of superintendent, doctors, nurses, and visitors and the external dignity of the state. A fine building, marble floors, and all that fiddle-faddle, making a good appearance, are impediments to the comfort of the destitute. As a rule, large debts ensue and pay-beds magically appear in the very place of the endowed beds given for non-paying need."

Lathrop was an early voice against experimentation on impoverished cancer patients, who never knew they were being used as guinea pigs. "Incurable cancer is now a matter of general and exhaustive study and the poor supply the principal material," she observed dryly. Once, in a letter, she described a woman who came to Saint Rose's from a nearby hospital, with much of her face destroyed by tumors and their treatment. "I suppose she is one of those whom they publish that they can cure," Lathrop commented. "I wish someone would stop those unstinted lies about cure which even that good hospital stoops to printing for the sake of attracting subjects for experiments."

Nothing about Rose Hawthorne Lathrop's early life would have pegged her to become a crusader for the dying. She was born in Lenox, Massachusetts, on May 20, 1851 — a year after her father published *The Scarlet Letter,* the novel of Puritan lust, sin, and guilt that made him famous. When she was two, the family moved to England and, a few years later, to Italy. On outings through Rome with her older brother, Julian, Rose discovered the visual and ritual splendor of the Catholic Church. It was a revelation for children from a Unitarian family. In hindsight, the experience seemed to plant the seeds for her future, but at the time she showed no inclination for a life of piety and charity. She was, in Julian's words, "an innate patrician," and "extremely fastidious" at that.

"Ugliness, dirt, disharmony revolted her and she averted herself from them with a hearty disgust," Julian wrote. She painted and wrote poetry. She loved romance and mischief. "She looked forward to the splendid carnival of human life, to a career in art, in society, to a bountiful and happy marriage."

A series of losses upended her life. Her father died the day before her thirteenth birthday. Her mother died when she was twenty. A few months later, against the wishes of her siblings, Rose married a struggling writer, George Lathrop. The union, tense from the start, grew rockier as Rose endured more loss: the death of her beloved sister and the estrangement of Julian, who feuded with George over the Hawthorne literary legacy. The Lathrop marriage stabilized after the birth of their son, Francis. But he died at age four, after a four-day bout of diphtheria, and the marriage teetered in grief.

Over the next decade, Rose and her husband struggled financially and lived apart for stretches, but together they studied Catholicism. Eventually, they converted, an event so stunning that fifty-six newspapers reported it. In the high-born society that Rose inhabited, Catholicism was viewed as the religion of immigrants and maids, and, worse, a faith built on the kind of ecclesiastic hierarchy and rigidity that had driven her Puritan ancestors to the New World. Rose never publicly explained why she converted. It did not save her marriage, but it changed her life.

She wanted to express her religious ideals by serving the most abject people imaginable. She concluded that nobody suffered more than people struggling with the dual cruelties of poverty and cancer. She received permission from the Church to leave her husband and pursue her mission.

Her brother regarded the act as martyrdom, if not madness. "Nothing less than the extreme would satisfy her thirst for self-sacrifice," he wrote. "Whatever was most abhorrent to the instincts of the flesh, that must she embrace; whatever was most hopeless and forlorn in human fate, that must she love and assuage."

Rose offered a less florid explanation near the end of her life, in an essay in the *New York Times Book Review and Magazine:* "As best I can, I am answering the question that has so often been put to me: Why in the

world did you set out to nurse this unat-
tractive disease?

"To tell the truth, I was shocked to discover how unusual my new endeavor
seemed to people — they seemed to be
acknowledging they were asleep in the
middle of a great disaster, that of the misery
of a class which they could so justly serve."

She went on to describe the death of her
close friend Emma Lazarus, the poet who
wrote those famous words inscribed on the
Statue of Liberty.

Give me your tired, your poor,
Your huddled masses yearning to breathe
    free,
The wretched refuse of your teeming shore.
Send these, the homeless, tempest-tost to
    me,
I lift my lamp beside the golden door!

The words captured Rose's mission, but she
brought up Emma Lazarus to make a different point: the world of difference between
dying amid privilege and dying in poverty.
Lazarus had died of cancer at age thirty-
eight, in the care of her family. "Though I
grieved deeply for her, I would not pity her,
for she never knew unaided suffering, but
every amelioration," Rose wrote. "On the

other hand, I finally heard of a case of abandonment to death which no one of any sensibility could ignore."

The story was of a young seamstress, unmarried and alone in New York City, and Rose heard it from a priest. Cancer had forced the woman to give up her job, tossing a respectable wage earner into poverty and eventually landing her on Blackwell's Island. Today that narrow strip in the East River, between Manhattan and Queens, is called Roosevelt Island, in honor of President Franklin D. Roosevelt. Reachable by the city's only sky tram, it has running tracks, river-view apartments, and a new inspirational monument dedicated to freedom. But in Rose's day the island was a human dumping ground that housed as many as 7,000 people at a time in forbidding institutions, including a penitentiary, a poorhouse, and the New York City Lunatic Asylum. The seamstress was not the only cancer patient to live her final days there. Not until 1909 did any of New York City's general hospitals admit people with cancer.

"Her despair was, most reasonably, complete," Rose wrote. "There was no one to stand forth and forbid the immolation of this woman upon the altar of fraternal indifference. A fire was then lighted in my heart to do something toward preventing such inhuman regulations for those who are too forlorn to protest."

In the summer of 1896, at age forty-five, Rose trained as a nurse at the New York Cancer Hospital (the nation's first hospital dedicated specifically to treating cancer and a forerunner of Memorial Sloan-Kettering Cancer Center). That September, she rented two tiny rooms near Manhattan's southern tip, scrubbed, painted, and supplied them with cots and bandages, and then set about recruiting cancer patients and women to help her care for them. At first, she treated patients in their homes, but she felt called to live among the sick, so she placed newspaper notices inviting patients to move in. In October 1896, Mary Watson, a sixty-five-year-old patient Rose had met in the hospital, took up the offer. Watson arrived thin and pale, wearing frayed bedroom slippers. Soiled bandages covered "half a face relinquished to the disease everyone abhorred," Rose observed. Watson had a bad cough, and every spasm crumpled her face with pain. Rose welcomed her, slept beside her to better care for her around the clock, and arranged for her burial seventeen months later.

Word got around, and Rose soon had

more patients than she could squeeze into two rooms. She rented a four-room apartment on nearby Water Street, facing the East River, where she housed up to six patients at a time and treated a never-ending parade of walk-ins in a cramped "relief room." Long before family-centered care would become a pillar of the hospice movement, grieving relatives also sought Rose's help. "Kind friend," her next-door neighbor, a Mrs. McNamara, wrote in a note on August 11, 1897. "The baby is dead. Can you oblige me with some kind of a little dress and old sheet?"

Many women responded to Rose's call for helpers, only to leave after a few days or months, repulsed by the odors and sights, worn out by the relentless labor, or dismissed because their work did not meet Rose's exacting standards. An exception was Alice Huber, a devout young Catholic from Kentucky who had come to New York to pursue art. She showed up at the apartment as a volunteer in late 1897 and, inspired by Rose's energy, stayed despite her revulsion. "I loathed everything about the place and still forced myself to dress a frightful sore that makes me sick to think of, even to this day," Huber later wrote.

Two events in the spring of 1898 proved

pivotal for Rose. Her estranged husband died, severing her only tie to the secular world, and Alice Huber moved in, providing Rose with a loyal partner in the work. In a display of devotion, Rose cut off her lustrous red hair and donned a makeshift habit — a dress of long, scratchy linen, a white neckerchief, and a simple cap resembling those worn by the Irish Sisters of Charity. (Alice copied the attire but kept her locks and wept for her shorn friend.)

A year later, Rose purchased the three-story brick house on Cherry Street that she named Saint Rose's, for Rose of Lima, the first canonized saint in the New World. She and Huber were accepted into the Third Order of Saint Dominic. Hawthorne took the name Mother Mary Alphonsa and Huber became Sister Mary Rose. In 1901, they founded a 100-bed facility, Rosary Hill, on lush rolling terrain twenty miles north of Manhattan.

Until she died in her sleep in 1926, Mother Alphonsa tried to rally support for the compassionate care of cancer patients and to dispel myths about the disease. She noted in letters that no Sister had fallen seriously ill from tending to patients. On this point too she was ahead of her time. Many people continued to believe that cancer was contagious even into the 1960s, when the hospice concept was introduced in America.

From 1930 through 1959, the Order she founded, the Dominican Sisters of Hawthorne, opened five homes modeled on the original two. Cicely Saunders knew of these facilities and wanted to learn more about their approach. During her first trip to the United States, in 1963, Saunders visited St. Rose's in Manhattan. The hulking five-story building bore no outward resemblance to the cozy brick townhouse of Rose Hawthorne Lathrop's days, which had been razed years earlier. But inside, Saunders found things operating much as they had from the start. St. Rose's closed years ago, but the Order still runs Rosary Hill. Sisters in white habits and black veils do all the nursing. Patients stay as long as necessary, in some cases years — for free.

Advanced Medicine, Delivered with the Kindness of the Human Heart

Cicely Saunders officially opened St. Christopher's Hospice on July 24, 1967, but she always considered the founding date to be February 25, 1948, when a forty-year-old cancer patient named David Tasma died.

In speeches and articles over the next half-century, Saunders often described their brief, intense relationship. She had been twenty-nine years old, a new social worker, when she met him on a hospital ward. Their conversations opened her eyes to the needs of dying patients, and his death taught her about the consuming grief of losing someone you love. Their relationship crystallized her life's mission, though the idea had been forming for years.

Saunders was born June 22, 1918, the eldest of three children in a wealthy, unhappy home. At age fourteen, tall, awkward, and shy, she was sent over her objections to an exclusive girls' school — and she was miserable. Years later, she would say that her sense of rejection, coupled with her parents' troubled marriage, inspired her empathy for the unfortunate and the outcast.

She enrolled in Oxford to study philosophy and economics but left to become a nurse at the start of World War II. An old back injury soon flared, making it impossible for her to lift or wheel patients, so she switched to medical social work. An agnostic from a family with no strong religious bent, Saunders had a revelation in the summer of 1945 and embraced evangelical Protestantism. With a convert's ardor similar to Rose

Hawthorne Lathrop's, Saunders began searching for a practical way to live out her religious ideals. As she recalled in a letter four decades later, "I asked what I had to do to say thank you and serve."

The answer came from David Tasma. He was a Jewish refugee from the Warsaw Ghetto, an agnostic, with no family and few friends in England, and he had inoperable cancer. He asked her if he was dying, and she told him yes. Late into the night, they used to wrestle with ineffable questions: What makes a life worthwhile? What matters at the end? What is it like to die? "David Tasma told me of the difficulties of laying down a life that felt incomplete and unfulfilled," she later wrote.

In a story she often told, Tasma once asked her for something to comfort him. She recited two psalms she knew and then offered to read more. "I only want what is in your mind and your heart," he replied. That simple desire came to represent everything she believed hospice should offer: the best therapies the mind could conceive along with the kindness, attention, and friendship of the human heart.

After Tasma died, Saunders decided to return to nursing as a first step toward creating that kind of hospice. A mentor, a surgeon, advised her to study medicine instead. "It is the doctors who desert the dying," he said. "There is so much more to be learned about pain and you will only be frustrated if you do not do it properly — and they won't listen to you."

While awaiting admission to medical school, Saunders volunteered at St. Luke's Hospital in London, which had been around since the 1890s, originally as St. Luke's Home for the Dying Poor. Her mentor proved to be right — pain and symptom management had a long way to go. She began to formulate principles that became the foundation of modern hospice care: respect for patients, scientifically based symptom control, and the belief that life can be lived even in the face of death. "I began to realize, as I listened to patients, that I was seeing something of their potential for making achievements of this part of their lives."

After earning her medical degree, Saunders tried to apply her skills and test her ideas at an old Sisters of Charity hospice in London, St. Joseph's. She loved the hardworking nurses but found the wards "virtually untouched by medical advance and support." She introduced the regular administration of drugs to control pain, vomiting, constipation, and anxiety, and she conducted research to validate and improve her methods. She pushed the nurses to keep scrupulous records and involve families in care. The effect was transformative. "Once Dr. Saunders came," recalled a nurse, Sister Mary Antonia, "it was like manna from heaven."

Florence Wald and the Groundswell for Change

Like Cicely Saunders and Rose Hawthorne Lathrop, Florence Wald found herself, in midlife, longing to find her life's mission. Hers was not a spiritual quest. She was an agnostic, the daughter of freethinkers ("My father's complaint was that the Church had taken too much money from people," she once said), and she would struggle for years to figure out how to create a hospice without a religious foundation. Instead, Wald's yearning for purpose sprang from the mix of idealism and discontent in the air in the 1960s. She was more than a generation older than the students marching for civil rights. As an Ivy League dean, she seemed to embody the establishment as campuses were erupting in protest against the Vietnam War. But she applauded those causes and sometimes joined the noisy demonstrations. She loved the blossoming spirit of dissent and wanted to shake things up in her field of nursing. Times were changing, and Wald believed the health care system should change with them. But how could she make that happen?

Cicely Saunders pointed the way. Her hospice approach gave concrete expression to Wald's thinking about how patients should be cared for throughout their lives, not just at the end. In hospice, Wald saw a proving ground for principles that she believed should apply to all health care: giving voice to patients, engaging families, getting professionals to work "collaboratively rather than competitively or antithetically." She envisioned a hospice groundswell as part of a broad movement to reform health care across the board — to change childbirth practices, improve care for seniors, humanize physician training, and relieve nurses of the administrative tasks that chewed their time so they could return to the bedside. Wald, five-foot-two, knew how to get things done — she had been instrumental in successfully fighting a move to shut Yale's nursing school a few years earlier. She realized she probably would not succeed in revolutionizing American health care, but surely she could get its first hospice off the ground.

She had been raised to challenge convention. Florence Sophie Schorske was born April 19, 1917, in New York City. Although she grew up in the straitlaced northern suburb of Scarsdale, her parents were card-carrying Socialists who carted their children to political rallies and debated the issues of the day at the dinner table. (Her older brother, Carl, would become a Pulitzer Prize-winning historian at Princeton.) At Mount Holyoke College, Florence studied physiology and sociology, the fusion of science and humanism that would run through her professional life. She earned a master's degree in nursing at Yale and worked with the Visiting Nurse Service of New York City, but she preferred research and teaching. She returned to Yale for a second master's degree, stayed on as an instructor, and became dean of nursing in 1958. An engineer named Henry Wald, who had been a subject in a research study she worked on during World War II — and who had proposed to her at the time, only to be rejected — read a newspaper article about her appointment and contacted her. By then he was a widower with two young children. They married in 1960, and he would become a partner in her hospice work.

Soon after she met Saunders, Wald resigned as dean to devote her energies to hospice. She and her family traveled to London in the summer of 1968, and Florence volunteered for a month at St. Christopher's. (Hospice champions from around the world would follow in her footsteps over the next quarter-century, trekking to St. Christopher's like pilgrims to Jerusalem. Saunders welcomed them, as long as they stayed a while and worked with patients.) After Wald returned home, she tapped three people to help her organize a hospice in New Haven — two pediatricians and a Yale chaplain. Soon a cancer surgeon, a nurse, and two more clergy signed on.

Their timing seemed perfect. In 1969, just as the group got down to work, psychiatrist Elisabeth Kübler-Ross published her blockbuster *On Death and Dying.* What had been a hushed topic when Saunders first came to Yale six years earlier now burst into public consciousness. Kübler-Ross had spent years studying the experience of dying through the eyes of patients. A tiny, commanding woman, she once stunned a room full of medical students at the University of Colorado by bringing in a teenager with terminal leukemia and interviewing the girl on the spot.

Her book gave searing accounts of the pain, emotional turmoil, and desolation of dying patients, and she put the blame on doctors and hospitals. A patient, she wrote, "may cry for rest, peace, and dignity, but he will get infusions, transfusions, a heart machine, or tracheotomy if necessary. He may want one single person to stop for one single minute so that he can ask one single question — but he will get a dozen people around the clock, all busily occupied with his heart rate, pulse, electrocardiogram, or pulmonary functions, his secretions or excretions, but not with him as a human being."

The technology had changed, but her criticism echoed Rose Hawthorne Lathrop's: Dying people want to be seen and heard. And they were neither in hospitals, where by the late 1960s most Americans died.

The work of Kübler-Ross set off a wave that spilled in many directions. Death studies became a hot topic in academia. "Death with dignity" organizations sprang up, forging a movement that shared the hospice goal of giving terminally ill patients more control over their lives but that advocated means that many hospice leaders refused to accept: euthanasia and physician-assisted suicide.

Around the country, small groups of nurses, clergy, social workers, and physicians came together, as Florence Wald's group had, to create alternatives to hospital care for dying patients.

"We had never heard of anything called hospice," said Hugh Westbrook, a Methodist minister who cofounded the first one in south Florida. "We were trying to make a difference for people nobody really cared about."

On November 19, 1971, Wald's group, by then forty strong, incorporated as a nonprofit and established an account at Orange National Bank with a $142.50 deposit. Although they named the organization Hospice, Inc., they privately referred to it as St. Christopher's in the Field. Henry Wald sold his engineering firm and enrolled in a master's program in architecture at Columbia University, with a focus on health facilities planning. For his thesis he drafted a blueprint for the hospice that his wife was determined to build — a place that would look and function much like the one in London.

But one aspect of the English model bothered the Connecticut group: religion. Like every place in history that had called itself a hospice, St. Christopher's was a Christian organization. Although it admitted patients regardless of faith and did not force prayer on anyone, Saunders insisted that medical care and spiritual care were inseparable at the end of life. Hospice without religion was unthinkable.

The Connecticut group by now included a Catholic priest, ministers of various Christian denominations, practicing Jews, Buddhists, New Age spiritual seekers, and nonbelievers like Florence Wald. Some members agreed that faith and God had to be integral to the care of dying patients. Others would have quit rather than establish a hospice on a religious footing. Still others set aside their beliefs to consider the issue strategically. Would the American public, far more diverse than England's, reject the hospice concept if it came shrouded in God? Would Medicare and health insurance plans cover it? Florence Wald knew that many people struggle spiritually as they face death, and she believed that hospice had to help them. But she defined spiritual care broadly. Hospice, she argued, should give patients the support that comes from their own religion or from art and music, from nature and poetry, from psychology or literature — in short, from any of the countless ways that humans find meaning.

The group spent long hours trying to reach consensus. Cicely Saunders, visiting from England, took part in one meeting and confessed that she felt torn. She liked the expansive definition of spiritual care, at least for the United States, because it might help hospice gain acceptance. Yet she did not see how a hospice could offer hope without Christianity — in particular, without holding out the possibility of resurrection. How else, she asked, would a doctor, a nurse, or a chaplain ease the terror of impending death?

In the end, Wald and her group endorsed spiritual care as a central tenet of hospice. They articulated a vision focused on "reverence for life" and "a purpose that is beyond us." The statement had a New Age ring typical of the era, but it marked a significant shift both for health care and the hospice movement. It affirmed that good care for terminally ill people extended beyond the bounds of medicine, and it established a humanist foundation for hospice. This would become the template for hospice in America.

With their mission spelled out, Wald and her group set out to make hospice a reality and promptly hit two walls: politics and money.

CHAPTER THREE:
CURE VERSUS CARE

"We believed in the idea so much we weren't prepared for the problems."

Nobody in those early years could have imagined today's hospice landscape.

Ninety-four percent of Americans live within an hour's drive of at least two hospice programs, and that's just on average. Some cities are saturated, and a family inclined to shop around (which few people do but everyone should) can find reviews on Yelp. Competition for dying patients sometimes turns nasty. Madison, Wisconsin, had one hospice for twenty-nine years, a nonprofit founded amid the fervor of the early hospice movement. In 2007, a second program opened. A third and fourth soon followed. Two of them wound up in court fighting about trademark infringement because both had logos with an illustration of a tree.

With hospices just about everywhere, it's

hard to imagine a time when the very word mystified people. "When we tried to get our first hospice off the ground and began asking people for support, everybody thought we were lisping 'hospital,' " recalled Mary McKenna, cofounder of the first hospice in Texas, in an interview with *Texas Monthly.*

Hospice is now a generic term, like Kleenex, but this implies that programs are all the same — that a hospice is a hospice is a hospice. In fact, the word covers a large universe. The Veterans Administration runs cutting-edge programs combining inpatient care, a huge home service, world-class research on palliative medicine, and physician training. There are hundreds of smaller nonprofit hospices, many of them decades old and beloved in their communities. Like the original hospice in Madison, many are losing ground to for-profit hospices.

The notion of investors profiting from hospices seemed blasphemous to Cicely Saunders and Florence Wald, when the first for-profit hospice opened in 1984. Yet by 2012, for-profit companies accounted for 60 percent of Medicare-certified hospice providers. The biggest player, VITAS Innovative Hospice Care, operated dozens of programs across eighteen states and the District of Columbia. The owner: Chemed

Corporation, a $1.3 billion company listed on the New York Stock Exchange and best known for its other holding, Roto-Rooter, of plumbing and sewer-cleaning fame.

Some of the early enemies of hospice, including hospitals, home health agencies, and nursing homes, now operate their own. So do seventy-five prisons, where inmates provide the bulk of the care. There are Catholic, Jewish, Presbyterian, Methodist, and Episcopal hospices. Shelby, Michigan, has a Muslim hospice; San Francisco and New York have Zen ones. Illinois, Georgia, and Pennsylvania have "green" hospices, with solar lighting and rain-collection barrels. A scattering of entrepreneurs sell "concierge" hospice to people willing to pay a premium for the promise of extra-special attention when the time comes. Some hospices run strictly on volunteer labor, grants, and donations, as they have from the beginning — they do not take Medicare or other reimbursement, so they do not have to abide by insurance rules. Even veterinarians have jumped on the hospice bandwagon, marketing pet hospice as an alternative to a high-dose barbiturate injection on a cold steel table.

Hospice gained public acceptance for the simple reason that it was a good idea.

"There was so much right about it, and so much that made sense about it to people," said Cynthia Adams, a nursing school administrator who has studied its history. But hospice grew because there was money in it. Medicare, the federal health insurance for people aged sixty-five and over, began covering hospice in 1983 and now pays the bills of 84 percent of patients in hospice care. Medicaid and private health insurance companies cover most of the remaining patients. For better and for worse, insurance coverage, Medicare especially, transformed a grassroots cause into an industry.

The flow of Medicare dollars carried programs farther, faster, than pioneers like Florence Wald ever dreamed, but with rules that have barely changed in thirty years — and that keep too many dying people from getting the services they need. While Medicare put hospices within geographic reach of just about everyone, it changed their essence. The ideal of care driven solely by the needs of patients collided with a system dictated by regulations and pressures to hold down costs. The success of hospice came with tradeoffs made from the start.

The fact that hospice succeeded at all is remarkable, considering how stubbornly the health care establishment resisted it. Florence Wald got her first taste of the battles to come on a Friday morning in May 1971, at a meeting with two high-level Connecticut health regulators, in Hartford, the state capital. She had gone there to find out how to obtain a license to operate the novel facility she intended to build.

The meeting began with one official asking, not in a welcoming way, "What does hospice mean?" He was a doctor. The other official said he had looked up the word in a dictionary, and the definition — "lodging for travelers" — puzzled him. What did that have to do with this agency, which regulated hospitals and nursing homes?

Wald gave them photographs from St. Christopher's, unfurled its blueprints, and said she wanted to open a similar facility. The doctor ignored the pictures of serene dying patients but noticed the specs on the blueprints for organ pipes and proudly told her that he played organ on Sundays in an inner-city church. That seemed to break the ice, but not for long. He challenged her: Connecticut already had plenty of beds for the sick in hospitals and nursing homes. Why add more? Why segregate the dying? Why create a new category of service for an already overburdened bureaucracy to monitor?

And what about "aggressive treatment"? Would Wald really deny desperately sick people the best that modern medicine offered?

She explained that the hospice would be aggressive in relieving pain and other symptoms and in providing emotional, spiritual, and practical support. He said he admired idealists but found her proposal "fuzzy" and difficult to grasp. After an hour and forty minutes, he showed her to the door.

"I wish you would go to a mountaintop somewhere," he said. "I might give you a lot of nuns, just so I don't have to be involved and see what you're doing."

Many hospice founders around the country faced similar hostility, or worse. Small groups of volunteers with no funding or clout faced off against nursing homes, hospitals, home health agencies, and their trade associations — big-budget operations with lobbyists, lawyers, and an abiding belief that their members already cared for dying patients just fine. Health care organizations sued Mary McKenna and three other volunteers working out of a church basement in Orange, Texas, to stop them from starting the first hospice in that state. Home health organizations — which served homebound patients, including the terminally ill, but at the time without a focus on pain management, spiritual support, or other hospice hallmarks — tried to shut down south Florida's first hospice, a tiny home service called Hospice of Miami. "They said we were practicing home health care without a license," recalled its cofounder, the Reverend Hugh A. Westbrook, "which in some sense was true."

Clergy, nurses, social workers, doctors, and true believers drove the early hospice efforts — it's likely there was not a marketer or a finance expert among them. They did not think of their projects as a competitive threat because they saw hospice as a mission, not a business proposition. Yet hospitals, nursing homes, and home health agencies recognized that a successful hospice program would lure away some of their most lucrative patients. Today, Medicare pays hospitals a predetermined rate for a patient with a given diagnosis, no matter how long a person stays, so the sickest patients who require lots of care are not necessarily the most profitable, and they can be money losers if they take up a bed too long. But in the early days of hospice, Medicare reimbursed hospitals separately for every service they provided — every tube of blood drawn, every aspirin administered, and every night the patient stayed. The more stuff a hospital did to patients and the longer it hung on to them, the sweeter the payday. And nobody had more stuff done to them, helpfully or not, than patients approaching the end of their lives, the very people hospice organizers intended to serve.

The health care establishment was not about to let go of these patients easily. There was more at stake than money — power and ego also came into play, as did honest disagreements about the limits of medicine and the role of doctors in caring for the very sick. Doris Howell, the children's blood specialist who had operated the slide projector for Cicely Saunders in a Philadelphia church and become a believer on the spot, eventually moved to the University of California, San Diego, where she broached the idea of developing a small hospice for children. Medical advances were dramatically improving the odds for children with cancer, especially leukemia. But doctors could not save every child. It troubled Howell to watch young patients blasted with powerful drugs that knocked them to the edge of death, and sometimes over it, while their parents were shoved into the background and given no information or support. "The part that was dropped all the time was the care of the family and the parents," she would say years later.

Howell invited the medical faculty to a meeting, served coffee and doughnuts, talked about the hospice concept, and suggested that San Diego, "with its open-mindedness," might be ready for this new approach. A pediatrician who happened to be Howell's former student popped out of her chair as if it were spring-loaded. "Under no circumstances will I ever send any child to hospice," she said. "I take care of my patients." As Howell stood in shocked silence, thinking, "But you don't," three more doctors declared that they would never make a hospice referral either.

Blinded by enthusiasm and politically naïve, many early hospice leaders had no idea how hard it would be to advance a new way to care for the dying. "We believed in the idea so much we weren't prepared for the problems," said Florence Wald.

Once Wald and her group realized the problems of licensing, financing, and building a place like St. Christopher's, especially in an antagonistic health care environment, they took a leap of faith and decided to care for dying patients at home instead. They had no proof it would work and no model to follow. Their guiding angel, Cicely Saunders, was just beginning to experiment with home hospice in England. But the Connecticut group also had no realistic alternative. A home service would require less capital and fewer layers of government approval than building a facility, and it would cost a lot less to operate than an inpatient program.

Although Wald agreed to this shift purely for pragmatic reasons, she promoted it as a matter of principle. At community meetings and in letters to the editor, she insisted that most patients *wanted* to die at home. In fact, she had no evidence to support the claim. She had interviewed dying patients for a research project a few years earlier and many had told her they preferred to die in their homes. But compared to what? Hospitals and nursing homes offered the only other options. No patient in her study had ever seen or probably even heard of a hospice.

Certainly some, maybe many people would opt to spend their final days at home no matter what. They would like sleeping on their lumpy old mattress or sitting in the shade of the trees they had planted to mark the birth of their children. They would prefer to have family members feed them ice chips and plump their pillows, rather than rely on rotating shifts of nurses and aides. But it was anyone's guess how many people would choose to die at home rather than in a beautiful, tranquil, full-service inpatient hospice like St. Christopher's, where trained staff, not an overwhelmed spouse or grieving daughter, labored around the clock. Saunders never considered providing home care until St. Christopher's was well established and had a waiting list longer than she would ever be able to accommodate inside the facility. She regarded the home service as an adjunct to, not a substitute for, inpatient care. The point of home care, like the point of everything she did, was to allow patients to determine how and where they would live until they died.

Florence Wald shared that view. Home hospice offered her an expedient foothold in a health care system that operated by different rules than England's, but she recognized the drawbacks. She worried especially about the huge demands on families. Doctors, nurses, aides, and social workers would visit, but the family would have to handle the unrelenting, messy, emotionally grueling work of caring for a loved one through death. Wald well knew that not all dying patients had families capable of dealing with the load. For that matter, not all patients had families or homes. While she publicly championed home hospice, privately she saw it as a defeat, and she despaired.

Cicely Saunders tried to cheer her up. "We are all so sorry that the thought of building has had to recede so far, but I am sure the home care will be an enormous success and comfort once it gets under way," Saunders wrote in her annual Christmas letter to Wald in 1973. "It really does get depressing though, doesn't it?"

Breaking Ground, At Last

Saunders turned out to be right about the success of home care. Hospice, Inc., later renamed Connecticut Hospice, enrolled America's first hospice patient in March 1974 and served eighty patients that first year. By the spring of 1975, it had a waiting list.

Wald and her group tried to stay true to their vision of comprehensive care, even within the confines of patients' homes. The initial staff included a doctor, two full-time registered nurses, three part-time licensed practical nurses, a social worker, a pharmacy consultant, and a coordinator of forty-six volunteers who visited patients, delivered supplies, and ran errands. Local clergy and several ordained members of the hospice board of directors provided spiritual care. All services were free.

The National Cancer Institute funded Hospice, Inc., the first of several dozen programs that the federal government would support with demonstration grants over the next few years. Soon there was talk in Washington of expanding Medicare to pay for hospice, and the demonstration projects were supposed to answer two questions. First, did hospice work — did patients really die in less distress? Second, and more importantly from Medicare's perspective, did hospice save money?

Under the $800,000 three-year grant to Hospice, Inc., patients had to have terminal cancer and a life expectancy, as the hospice's 1975 annual report put it, of "weeks, not months or years." Although these were the sorts of patients the founders had always envisioned serving, nobody until then had defined strict criteria for eligibility or imposed a time frame on life expectancy. The question of who qualified for hospice care — and who did not — would become more important when Medicare and insurance companies began to pay for it.

As the Connecticut hospice evolved from a band of crusaders into a functioning program, conflicts brewed and eventually exploded. After state officials twice rejected applications to build and operate an inpatient facility, the board of directors hired an executive with an MBA, Dennis Rezendes, to break the logjam. He knew how to steer a project through the regulatory maze but not how to get along with the steel-willed Florence Wald. She found him bossy and arrogant. He said she micromanaged and second-guessed his every move. While she was away on vacation in August 1975, he wrote to the board complaining of "the tensions created by her, the additional work burden imposed on some of us, the meddling in the affairs of other departments, and the creation of doubts and the seeming never-ending countermanding of directions." The staff was in shambles.

Rezendes gave the board an ultimatum: She must go or he would. The turmoil reached a peak that fall, and the board asked for Wald's resignation. She submitted it, then immediately withdrew it. The board voted unanimously to fire her.

On the surface, the fight looked like a garden-variety workplace power struggle. But on a deeper level, it illustrated an emerging clash between principles and pragmatism in the hospice movement — a conflict that has shaped the system we have today. Wald felt devastated by her dismissal and received heartfelt letters from supporters, including Cicely Saunders and Elisabeth Kübler-Ross. (A few years later, Wald would return to the movement as passionate as ever, leading efforts to establish hospices in prisons.) Meanwhile, Rezendes convened the first national symposium on hospice care, in Connecticut, the day after Wald's firing. In a rousing speech, he cheered the growing movement and its spirit of cooperation.

Rezendes soon obtained state approval for a building. The first hospice facility in this country broke ground on November 20, 1977, a sunny Sunday afternoon. Twelve hundred people, among them hospice patients in wheelchairs and Wald herself, attended the ceremony. It began with an ecumenical service of thanksgiving and hope. The site spanned six acres of a former cow pasture in Branford, a quaint town eight miles east of New Haven, on Long Island Sound.

The $3.6 million building would have forty-four beds. The hospice already cared for at least twice as many patients at home on an average day, which meant that the inpatient facility would serve as an adjunct to the home service, not the other way around. The inpatient service would admit the patient who needed to be stabilized or whose pain raged out of control or whose family wobbled dangerously on an emotional cliff and needed a few days' respite. But most hospice patients would never step inside.

Building a facility marked a proud achievement for the Connecticut group and a milestone for the movement. But the hospice model in America had already been set, and it was home care.

While officials in Connecticut ceremonially shoveled clods of soil, more than 100 grassroots groups in thirty-two states were planting the seeds for hospices in their communities. Many groups, like Wald's, brought together nurses, chaplains, doctors, and social workers — people from health care who wanted to bring good science and medicine to bear on the compassionate care of dying patients. But some groups came to hospice from far outside the health care establishment, with an Age of Aquarius aura. In hospice they saw a way to fuse self-help, mysticism, and metaphysics, and to liberate the dying process from the heavy-handed control of health care professionals.

For all their high-mindedness, the more mainstream groups did not always appreciate their free-spirited comrades in the movement. "You don't know how many New Age flakes you would meet," recalled Madalon Amenta, former executive director of the Hospice Nurses Association (now the Hospice and Palliative Nurses Association) and author of the first nursing textbook on care for the terminally ill. "I didn't know how they could find their way from the house to the office."

Among the fledgling hospice groups in those days was one in Florida organized by Hugh Westbrook. More than anyone else, he would turn the struggling, idealistic movement into today's multibillion-dollar industry.

The Humble Beginnings of a Hospice Empire

Westbrook knew nothing about Florence Wald or Cicely Saunders when he got the idea of starting a program to care for dying patients in their homes. He had worked as a hospital chaplain on cancer wards in the late 1960s, while finishing his studies at Duke Divinity School, and he saw the need.

Over the next seven years, he moved from one Methodist ministry to another, in North Carolina and then Florida, butting against church authorities over his outspoken support for school busing and gay rights. He had a wife and young children to support, and he cobbled together several part-time jobs, including co-teaching a course on death and dying at the local junior college, with Esther Colliflower, a registered nurse. "We weren't that good at teaching or research, so we decided to try to take care of people," he would say years later.

Westbrook and Colliflower badgered a local cancer specialist to refer patients. Finally a patient named Emmy Philhour called them. "She said, 'If you take care of me so I don't have to go to the hospital and I can remain at home, I will teach you what to do,' " Colliflower recalled recently. She and Westbrook learned the rudiments of hospice by following Philhour's leads, caring for her and supporting her and her husband in all the ways they asked. For Colliflower, the experience became a guide for patient-directed end-of-life care.

After Philhour died, Westbrook and Colliflower found another patient and then another — they could not handle more than one or two at a time. In 1978, they incorporated their venture as the nonprofit Hospice of Miami. When home health agencies tried to get it shut down for operating without a license, Westbrook took up a new cause. He started lobbying for a state law to license hospices and to define them as a distinct health care category, independent of hospitals, nursing homes, and, needless to say, home health agencies.

Westbrook went to Tallahassee, the capital, to see a friend who had just been elected to the legislature. Carrie Meek, the granddaughter of slaves (and later a five-term representative in Congress) had also co-taught seminars with Westbrook at the junior college (today's Miami Dade College). On a yellow legal pad, Westbrook jotted down the provisions of the law he wanted. Colliflower and a chaplain outlined the clinical components of good end-of-life care. With the help of Meek, other contacts, and Westbrook's considerable charm, those scribbles would come fairly close to the Florida law passed just before the close of the 1979 legislative session.

It was the nation's first law to recognize hospice, establish criteria for eligibility, and set standards for care. Under the law, patients had to have a life expectancy of one year or less, and programs had to offer comprehensive services, including medical, nursing, and psychosocial support. "It couldn't just be handholding," Westbrook said.

The law required hospices to operate as nonprofits and accept patients regardless of their ability to pay. Westbrook had pushed hard for these provisions, in large part to protect low-budget ventures like his from being swallowed by large health care companies. He would later say that in his wildest dreams, he never imagined that one day he would become the industry giant.

For years after his first successful foray into lobbying, Westbrook made it all sound so simple — an affable young minister walking the halls of power, chatting up lawmakers, making friends, and selling the hospice idea. His strongest, most unlikely ally was a health care executive named Donald Gaetz, who had recently moved to Florida to open a hospital-based hospice. Gaetz started out opposing Westbrook's bill but, once the two men sat down, Westbrook won him over. Gaetz quit his job and they teamed up.

They were poles apart politically — Westbrook was a liberal firebrand, Gaetz a conservative Republican. (He would go on to serve in the Florida Senate and as its president in the 2013–2015 session.) But they shared a view of what good hospice care looked like. And they agreed that Medicare had to pay for it, or hospice would not survive.

Most hospices relied on donations and served patients for free. In 1980, the federal government selected twenty-six programs, including Hospice of Miami, to participate in a two-year hospice demonstration project. The programs received reimbursement for their costs, which provided a financial cushion and fueled their growth. Westbrook, Colliflower, and now Gaetz went from serving a couple of patients at a time to ten or twenty. They opened a second nonprofit. Colliflower visited St. Christopher's in England to learn from Cicely Saunders.

But where would money come from when the demonstration project ended? Westbrook and Gaetz saw Medicare as the only feasible, sustainable revenue source. Most hospice patients were sixty-five and over. Medicare paid their bills if they died in a hospital — why shouldn't it pay if patients chose hospice? Westbrook and Gaetz also assumed, correctly, that once Medicare covered hospice, Medicaid and private insurance plans would follow.

Westbrook hauled out the yellow legal

pads again. With help from Connecticut's Dennis Rezendes, Westbrook and Gaetz began putting together a bill, modeled on the Florida law, creating a Medicare hospice benefit.

They ran into stiff opposition, and not only from the usual suspects in the health care industry. The hospice movement itself was divided on the question of Medicare coverage. Many hospice organizers agreed that hospice would wither away, a fringe idea that never took hold, without legitimacy and money from Medicare. At least as many people argued that Medicare's voluminous rules and regulations would compromise, if not destroy, the expansive hospice movement and its patient-centered ethic. Milestone or millstone? Hospice leaders fought about it for years.

Both sides would turn out to be right.

On March 25, 1982, the House of Representatives Committee on Ways and Means held hearings on legislation to authorize a Medicare hospice benefit. Forty-two people testified. Written statements came in from dozens of organizations representing hospitals, physicians, psychiatrists, nurses, hospices, dance therapists, volunteers, clergy, psychodrama practitioners, physical therapists, insurance companies, and more. Congress had taken up a Medicare hospice bill before. It would pass that year with strong bipartisan support. Most hospice leaders had come around too, though some remained wary.

Looking back from the twenty-first century — when a partisan furor (and nonsense about death panels) erupted over a proposal by President Obama to allow Medicare to reimburse doctors for time they spent simply discussing end-of-life options — it is almost impossible to imagine how the hospice benefit made it through Congress. It was the only new health service entitlement created during President Ronald Reagan's first term. It also was the only Medicare benefit crafted not only to improve patient care but also to cut government spending. In the end, advocates convinced lawmakers that hospice care would be cheaper for Medicare than paying for the aggressive treatment that so many patients received up until they died.

Research would prove the point years later, but at the time, the evidence was preliminary at best. Yet Congress focused so intently on the potential cost savings that one expert — who had been summoned to testify on this very issue — urged lawmakers to concentrate on best practices instead of the price of end-of-life care. "I am somewhat distressed that the cost premise has been so prominent in the rationale for hospice," he said.

Just as Hugh Westbrook had argued, Medicare coverage helped hospice grow and thrive. And just as other hospice leaders had feared, Medicare dollars and dictates altered an altruistic cause, creating a bureaucratic and increasingly profit-driven enterprise. The only surprise was that the biggest beneficiaries turned out to be Westbrook and his partners. As soon as the Medicare benefit went into effect, they opened the first for-profit hospice. In the years ahead, they would build it into the VITAS chain — a story we'll get to in Chapter 12.

The Medicare hospice benefit has not changed substantively since day one, and on the positive side, it honors founding ideals of the movement. The law requires hospices to provide a broader array of services than any other type of health care provider is bound to offer, a nod to the principles of holistic, comprehensive care. In addition to medical supervision and nursing, Medicare-certified hospices must provide spiritual and social work support for families as well as for patients. Hospices also must offer bereavement services. In another unique provision aimed at preserving the spirit of the early movement, Medicare requires hospices to utilize volunteers.

On the down side, Medicare rules create barriers for people who need services. To be eligible, a patient must be doctor-certified to have a life expectancy of six months or less if the primary disease runs its normal course. (This marked a downgrade from the one-year prognosis under the Florida law Westbrook had pushed, one of several money-saving compromises.) Hospices do not have to drop a patient who lives longer than six months, but doctors must re-certify eligibility. All this causes two big problems for patients. First, oncologists, heart specialists, kidney specialists, and other physicians who treat seriously ill patients cannot always say with certainty when that six-month clock starts ticking — and making the call has become more difficult because there is always another drug or procedure to try. Everyone in medicine knows of patients who seemed on the verge of death, only to bounce back against all odds. The six-month rule has too often served as a dodge, a way for patients and doctors alike to put off hospice until a later day, and put it off again until it's too late.

The second problem is that, if a hospice does its job well, the patient may stabilize and even improve. Since Medicare scrutinizes extensions, especially if the patient is not deteriorating, the patient may wind up being discharged from the program that's keeping her alive.

The paperwork required to certify and recertify patients for hospice has grown thicker over the years and consumes significant chunks of doctor and nurse time. In researching this book, we observed a doctor spend eight hours over the week — a full day, essentially — reviewing the charts of patients, reading the notes of the nurses who admitted them, and signing off on forms called Initial Certification of Terminal Illness. Doctors of course should approve hospice admissions, but at least one-quarter of the patients had already died by the time their paperwork reached this physician's desk. Still she had to explain in detail why she deemed them terminal. One day, after three of these in a row, she sighed in exasperation and sang a few notes from "Ding Dong! The Witch Is Dead," from *The Wizard of Oz:*

As coroner I must aver, I thoroughly examined her.

And she's not only merely dead; she's really most sincerely dead.

Patients (or their families) also have to deal with Medicare paperwork upon hospice enrollment, and the form that gets the most attention requires them to agree to forego coverage for potentially curative treatments. Nobody is forced into hospice, and patients retain the right to pay on their own for curative care if they want it — they simply must acknowledge that Medicare will not foot the bill for it while they are on hospice. But this rule throws up enormous psychological and practical barriers for patients. It sets up hospice as a stark choice between the possibility of cure, however remote, and compassionate care. It is probably the biggest reason why more people who could benefit from hospice stay away.

"There's a dichotomy, and it sounds like hospice is the booby prize," said Elizabeth Menkin, a longtime hospice physician. "Nobody wants the booby prize. Everybody wants the miracle."

The Medicare benefit ended any prospect for comprehensive inpatient programs like St. Christopher's in England. The regulations limit how much of a hospice's Medicare charges can go to inpatient care, and through a complicated formula, the rules

102

also limit the average payment per patient. Essentially, eighty cents of every dollar that a hospice charges Medicare must be spent providing home care. As a result, hospice in America is far from the all-compassing service that Florence Wald envisioned. "As a caring concept, hospice is wonderful," said Marsha Hurst, a research scholar at Columbia University's Institute for Social and Economic Research and Policy. "As a health care benefit, hospice is not that wonderful."

Nurses, doctors, aides, and the rest of the hospice team come to the house (or the nursing home, board-and-care facility, or wherever the patient lives), often providing the best care the patient will ever receive. But the hospice system made all of us responsible for helping the people we love to die well.

Nothing we will ever do is more demanding. It can also be profoundly rewarding. That often comes as the biggest surprise about the hospice experience. And it did for Nat Landes, age ninety-two, who agreed to hospice for his wife only after months of saying no.

■ ■ ■ ■

PART TWO:
THE PATIENTS

■ ■ ■ ■

CHAPTER FOUR:
EVELYN LANDES: HOUSE CALLS

"We had a helluva good year."

Soon after starting on hospice care, Evelyn Landes turned ninety but was too weak and confused to celebrate. A year later, she greeted guests, including her hospice doctor, at her birthday party. The following month, she took a half-hour drive to attend her granddaughter's baby shower. She talked about wanting to meet her first great-grandchild.

That Evie was still alive surprised everyone. That she could take any pleasure in her family and friends was almost unfathomable.

Before starting on hospice she had been gravely ill with congestive heart failure. Episodes of dementia were robbing the large, boisterous family of the intuitive, impish soul who showered love on five grandchildren. After repeated bouts of pneumonia, Evie had been given a week or two to live. A doctor in the hospital suggested hospice.

Evie's husband, Nat, got angry. Whatever the doctor said and however he said it, Nat heard it to mean, "She's old, let her go. Let hospice warehouse her at home." As long as Evie had the capacity to engage in life, to look forward to anything, Nat wanted to keep her alive. He never imagined that hospice would turn out to be the best way possible to do that.

Running Downhill

Heart disease ran in Evie's family. It debilitated her father, killing him in middle age. Her brother also had died from chronic heart failure. She took her genetics seriously and went to a heart health program at Sequoia Hospital, a regional center for cardiac care in the San Francisco Bay Area. She got a treadmill and used it. She watched her diet, had two angioplasties, and took vitamins, supplements, and medications for high blood pressure and cholesterol.

Nat, an engineer by training and temperament, devised a spreadsheet of all the pills she was taking — twenty-five a day at one point. He noted the company name, generic name, dosage, prescription number, renewal date, and side effects. And there were plenty of side effects, from constipation to confusion.

Evie had problems chewing and swallowing, so that bits of food and liquid backed up in her lungs, causing repeated episodes of life-threatening pneumonia. Terrifying trips to the emergency department at Sequoia Hospital came closer together.

Nat and Evie were lucky that their four children lived in the Bay Area and that Nat, into his nineties, remained robust — amazingly healthy except for what he jokingly called "the usual aging of the parts." He and Evie had visited many friends in nursing homes and felt the same way about institutional care: no. They had made a pact on that.

But the demands of home care were relentless, from getting Evie in and out of bed to running to the store for groceries. For stretches of time on many days, he was in constant motion between the kitchen and the living room and the bedroom — adding or subtracting medications, trying to get his wife to eat, and knowing that the one thing he could count on was that whenever he sat down he would have to get up. Looking back, he would say, "It was like working in a factory." He hired private caregivers.

Evie's condition continued to deteriorate. She suffered from dehydration, painful swelling in her legs, drug side effects that affected her balance and kidneys, and her own frustration at her loss of control. Totally out of character, she sometimes screamed when certain people came near.

In January 2010, another pneumonia emergency brought Evie to Sequoia Hospital. Nat spoke with a hospitalist, the physician whose job is to coordinate care for hospital patients. The doctor mentioned hospice, and Nat lost his temper, feeling he and his wife were simply being dismissed. It was not the first time someone had broached the possibility of hospice — a family member had brought it up months earlier, and Nat had reacted with anger then too.

The day after the conversation with the hospitalist, Nat spoke with another doctor. She treated him more like an equal, with respect. She said: Your wife is terribly ill. Yes, she may die in a week, but it also may be months. The doctor did not instantly change Nat's mind about hospice — he was determined to manage his wife's care. But she gave him hope that whatever time was left to Evie could be worth living.

Nat finally agreed to hospice several

months later, and what followed defied all his expectations and assumptions (not to mention her doctors' prognoses). "We had a helluva good year," he said.

When Nat Met Evie

Both creative and smart, Nat and Evie had their differences in sixty-eight years of marriage. The differences began at birth, she very poor, in Willows, in rural Northern California, he in New York City. She was an artist and teacher who longed for a Camelot kind of life. He was a civil engineer with a long career in the military. At their house in the San Francisco Bay Area, floor-to-ceiling bookcases reflected their left brain/right brain split: art and fiction on Evie's side, history and science on Nat's.

He first caught sight of her in a classroom at the start of World War II. Nathan Landes was stationed at Fort Ord, in Monterey, California. Concerned that so many soldiers were illiterate, he and a couple of other officers suggested bringing in local schoolteachers. Beautiful Evelyn Zemel was one of them.

That she was the only Jewish teacher and he was the only Jewish officer did not escape the notice of the Jewish Welfare Board, a group of local women who helped soldiers find places to go for Jewish holidays and events. Nat resisted being fixed up, a fit of pride he later regretted. As he put it, "I lost out on a year of knowing her!" When finally they did meet, at another officer's birthday party, he fell hard. Although it took her a bit longer, Evie did, too. When they decided to marry, in 1943, Evie asked her principal for three days off. He refused and said she would lose her job if she left. Evie left anyway.

After the war, Nat got work with a builder. He eventually founded a construction company and built a large house in the redwoods for their four children.

The do-it-yourself mentality came naturally to Evie and Nat. He served as mayor of his town, Woodside, during a high-growth era and as the president of their synagogue. He also served almost forty years in active and reserve military duty. Evie went back to college in her mid-forties, earned a master's degree in art education, taught textile arts at the college level, and founded a quilters guild. After their kids were grown, Nat built another house, and he and Evie moved in. This one showcased Evie's needlepoint and extraordinary quilts, with a large room for her equipment and supplies. When showing a visitor around the house, Nat stopped to admire one of his favorites of Evie's quilts — a geometric sampler used for teaching. "It has all these different patterns, but they fit," he said, gently fingering the material. "The more you look, the more you see."

What Good Hospice Care Looks Like

On June 26, 2010, the Landeses signed up for hospice with Pathways Home Health & Hospice, a large nonprofit operating in the Bay Area since 1977. Hospice nurses would come at least twice a week, and home health aides would come several times a week to bathe and dress Evie and change the bedding. The doctor would come every six weeks.

When Ellen Brown, medical director of Pathways, first met her, Evie had just been in the hospital again and had a lot of delirium. The doctor and Nat went over the spreadsheet of medications, as they would at every visit. She stopped the iron pills and the cholesterol drug Lipitor that Evie had been taking for years. Iron was constipating and she was not anemic, nor did they need to worry about high cholesterol. Brown also eliminated the blood pressure medicine hydralazine, which she thought might have contributed to Evie's episodes of delirium, and made other drug adjustments. The

113

upshot of all these changes was that Evie was more clear-headed and mobile than she had been in a long time.

Even with hospice support, Nat juggled people coming and going. He got impatient when things did not work the way he knew they should, and could lose his temper when he pointed it out and was brushed off as a ranting old man. The mechanics of hospital beds drove him nuts — he was an engineer, after all — and he spent a lot of time arguing with the bed-supply company. The first bed sent over for Evie had railings too thin for her to grip. The second one had a gap between the railings and the mattress and Nat feared that she might slip through. "Come get this bed now or I'm putting it out on the street," he demanded — only to be told that Medicare did not cover the kind of bed he wanted. Pathways got Evie the right bed, and straightened out a problem with the oxygen equipment.

Nat had nothing but praise for the hospice care itself. Having run a business, he appreciated how well the hospice staff worked together and with his wife, and how they paid attention to him. "It's unusual to find that many wonderful people in a company," he said. "From Doctor Brown, a thoughtful, caring, and loving person, to the nurse in the office, who if she didn't know the answer she got it or sent someone, to aides who came to bathe my wife, change her diapers, fix her nails, fix her hair, whatever made her feel better. My wife — from when she was mentally alert to delirious — was happy to see them when they came into the house. When she saw them, she had a big smile on her face."

It helped immeasurably that Nat had the resources to employ two loving caregivers. And when Medicare rules got complicated, delaying the release of supplies or medications that Evie needed, Nat went out and bought them. Still, the support that Pathways provided cannot be understated. The hospice advised him on every aspect of caring for Evie, down to making sure he used distilled water in the oxygen concentrator so that minerals wouldn't clog up the tubes. Like his wife, Nat always was happy when people from Pathways came over.

"What Questions Do You Have for Me?"

One morning nearly a year into Evie's hospice care, her doorbell rang, and there stood Ellen Brown and Elsie Gyang, a fourth-year medical student at Stanford University. Twice a month except in summer, Brown took a medical student on her rounds. She knew the Landes family well. She knew not to schedule a home visit on a Wednesday, because Evie's quilting group came that day. Brown greeted the caregiver, Olga, by name. Olga led them past the baby grand piano that Evie used to play and through the hall draped with multi-colored quilts that Evie made.

In the high-ceilinged family room, big windows and a skylight let in views of flowering vines and potted succulents. A wisp in a nightgown, Evie occupied very little space on a deep leather couch. A clear tube ran from her nose around her head to the oxygen machine plugged into the wall.

Brown sat in the chair closest to Evie. "Sounds like you're sleeping better."

"I am," Evie said.

"Are you able to get outside and enjoy your garden?"

"Yes, I get out for an hour, a half-hour." Evie touched the arm on the couch and looked out the window.

The questions followed quickly but in a certain progression:

"Coughing?"

"Yes."

"Coming up?"

"Yes."

"What does it look like?"

"Gunk."

"Fevers?"

"Not as far as I know."

"What did you have for breakfast?"

"Fruit."

"How is your appetite?"

"Oh, I can always eat." A small laugh.

"Do your quilting friends come by?"

They talked a little about quilting, but hadn't gotten to what Brown knew was really bothering Evelyn. "What questions do you have for me?" she asked Evie.

"I want to get rid of this thing," Evie said, meaning the tube in her nose. She said she'd tried not wearing it, when going to the bathroom.

"What don't you like about it?" Brown asked.

"I don't want to wear it."

"Is it how it feels or how it looks?"

"Both."

"It's hard on your face," Brown agreed, but added, "It's possible if we take it off your breathing will get a lot worse." She paused and looked into Evie's eyes. "I'm giving you a choice. It's not a good choice."

While Evie pondered the choice, Nat announced his entrance with a booming, "Hi, Tootsie!" to his wife. Introduced to Gyang and told they'd been discussing the oxygen machine, he looked from the two doctors to his wife and immediately changed his tone of voice. "In twenty minutes you're gasping for breath," he said to Evie, kindly. "If we had another way, the doctor would be doing it."

Brown resumed with Evie. "So you're enjoying food?"

No answer.

"Sleeping?"

"Pretty good."

"What would you like to be doing?"

No answer. Nat put in, "She loves friends coming over, and kids. Sometimes when they come she says no. I try. She got her hair fixed up a week ago."

Brown turned back to Evelyn. "I know your appearance is very important. Do you feel you get to decide when people visit?"

Before Evie could answer, Nat put in a joke: "There's only one thing you're not going to have control over, and that's me!" Brown made sure Evie had time to answer for herself. She smiled.

After an hour and fifteen minutes with the Landeses, the doctors were back in the car. Gyang told Brown she'd always wondered why hospital patients complained so much about nostril tubes. They seem so light and flexible. Now Gyang said, "I see how it could be very annoying."

The medical student was surprised by her first hospice patient. "She looked pretty good to me, from what I had pictured in my head," she told Brown.

"If she continues to improve, I don't know," Brown said, partly in humor and partly in a nod to Medicare reality, "I may have to take her off hospice."

"Let's Go for a Ride!"

While the goal of hospice is not to prolong life but to maximize the quality, research now shows that hospice may increase the longevity of terminally ill patients. The largest study of its kind compared the survival rates of 4,493 Medicare patients. On average, those on hospice lived twenty-nine days longer. Patients with congestive heart failure, like Evie, did particularly well. They lived an average of eighty-one days longer than non-hospice patients with the same diagnosis. This is particularly significant because many people think of hospice as mainly for cancer patients. That was true in the early days of hospice, but now fewer than 40 percent of hospice patients have cancer as a primary diagnosis. More than 11 percent of hospice patients in 2011 had terminal heart disease. Like Evie, many may do badly for a while and then stabilize.

She stayed on hospice fifteen months, often able to walk again and breathe without pain. She knew she had dementia, but when a hitch occurred, she could say, "I can't remember!" and laugh at herself. At one point, a hospice nurse wrote on Evie's chart: "pleasantly confused," meaning that she may not know what day it was, but she was cheerful and not agitated. Evie and Nat went to the beach instead of the hospital.

Nat knew it was going to be a very good day when Evie got up in the morning and said, "Let's go for a ride!" They covered a lot of Northern California, west to the beach at Half Moon Bay and south to the redwoods in the Santa Cruz Mountains. They would drive for two hours to one of Evie's favorite nurseries, where she would spend an hour, at first with a walker and then in a wheelchair, seeing and smelling the native flowers and shrubs that she loved and had planted all around her house. She knew all the species and varieties.

The family moved more potted plants and bird feeders around to the patio outside Nat and Evie's bedroom, so she could still watch the birds when she could not get out of bed.

Evie's quilting group came every Wednesday, working in the large room built just for this purpose, with a 14-foot-wide sewing machine, work tables, and exquisitely labeled and organized plastic bins. Some days Evie could join the group only for a minute or two, and sometimes she was too ill to leave the bedroom, but they always came.

Evie and Nat's grandchildren visited too. One came all the way from Israel and spent a long time by Evie's side. Just around her one-year mark on hospice care, Evie attended the baby shower of her oldest grandchild, Beth Landes Fishman. Evie had never been subtle about her hopes on this score. A few years earlier, before Beth was even thinking about a baby, Evie had given her a copy of *Goodnight Moon,* inscribed: "I read this to all my children. Read it to yours." Now photos of Beth, with radiant face and swollen belly, joined the many pictures of bar and bat mitzvahs, graduations, and weddings on display in the Landeses' home.

After Rebecca was born, that August, her photos took their place among the others. Evie talked about meeting the baby. Beth lived 350 miles away, in the Los Angeles area. She planned to fly up with Rebecca at the end of October, to spend the last few weeks of her maternity leave with her family and introduce Evie to her first great-grandchild.

■ ■ ■ ■

By mid-October, Evie was very ill. She told at least one family member that she wanted to die. She stopped eating and became alternately agitated and unresponsive. It seemed unlikely that she would make it until the end of the month, but Beth could not take the baby on a trip until she got her immunizations at eight weeks old.

As the eight-week mark approached, Evie was fading but still had moments of responsiveness. She welcomed a chaplain from Pathways, and was calm and peaceful when he left. Told that Beth and the baby were coming the next day, she squeezed her daughter, Debbie's, hand, though what that meant was anybody's guess.

It usually takes six hours to get from Beth's house to her parents' house, and thirty minutes more to Evie and Nat's. But traveling with an infant slows things down, with breaks to nurse and change diapers. It was getting dark when Rebecca woke, near Salinas, and Beth turned off the freeway to stop and feed her but got stuck in hellacious Friday night traffic. Rebecca screamed for the last forty-five minutes of the trip. They finally made it to Beth's parents' house, late at night. On the phone, Nat said Evie was sleeping and they should wait until morning to come.

When they arrived at the house around eleven a.m., along with Beth's sister, Marni, and their mother, Joyce, Evie had no color and lay absolutely still. Beth, a physical therapist, had worked with critically ill people but this sight shocked her. To Marni, Evie looked liked she'd already died.

Joyce said, "Why don't we put some clothes on, and you can hold the baby?" No response. They got her dressed and gently placed Rebecca across her chest. Evie moved a hand and smiled slightly. Somebody helped her touch Rebecca, and they took a picture. When they picked up the baby and took turns holding her, Evie turned her head to follow the sound.

She died that night.

Beth and Marni are sure that their grandmother hung on because she wanted to meet her great-grandchild. For some in the Landes clan, this would become family lore, and it would appear in her death notice in the *San Francisco Chronicle,* alongside an old photo of the dark-haired young beauty who'd once defied her boss to go off and get married: "Evie passed on at her home in Woodside following a long illness, just hours after meeting and getting to hold her first great-grandchild."

Other family members say the idea that Evie controlled the timing this way — or even that she registered the baby's presence — is pure fantasy. She had not eaten in ten days. Yes, her heart was beating but in all the ways that mattered, she was already gone.

Ellen Brown says it's impossible to know why people die when they do. She has seen other instances of remarkable timing. For all that hospice has revealed about the mechanics of dying and the needs of people going through it, on its deepest level, the process remains mysterious.

Nat knows only that his wife wanted to meet the baby, and that his granddaughters believe Evie waited for Rebecca. To which he quips: "Had I known, I would've said, 'Why don't you stay away another week?' "

CHAPTER FIVE:
ALICE AND YING WUN:
A FRAGILE FAMILY PEACE

*"The end of life is like an earthquake.
You just don't prepare."*

One day, apparently out of the blue, Alice Wun had trouble talking. Two days later, the sixty-eight-year-old mother of seven had a diagnosis of terminal cancer, and her family was huddled in the hospital waiting room, trying to decide what to do. Her sleepless husband, Ying, was too stunned to speak.

The family had not been in the same room together for a long time, and they were not all there yet. Two of Alice and Ying's daughters and two sons had gathered, with Jeanne, the eldest daughter, running between her mother, her father, the doctors, and her siblings to relay information — the ambassador role she had always played in the family. Another brother and sister would arrive soon. One brother had not been seen in twenty years, and nobody expected that to change now. It would be hard for any family to overcome the shock of such a devastating diagnosis and think clearly, and even harder for a frayed family. It was especially tough for a family that had never talked about dying, let alone planned for it. Before the day was over, the siblings would learn that Alice and Ying did not even have a will.

Now the siblings argued. Their mother wasn't old and she had seemed so healthy. Wasn't surgery worth a try? What about chemo and radiation first, to shrink the tumor? Why not throw everything at it? But surgery would be brutal. And, even if she could survive it after doctors removed whatever cancer they could, then she would face chemotherapy and radiation, with debilitating side effects.

Alice had already told Jeanne she wanted to go home. Ying was totally opposed. "Who will care for her?" he asked, knowing it would not be him. And he had another concern: "We can't have her die at home. How am I going to sell the house?" In China, everyone knew the *feng shui* rules to rid the house of negative energy. In this country, people did not understand and would be scared off from buying a house in which death had occurred.

But Alice knew what she wanted, and the family had to honor it. They did not "choose" hospice — not in the sense that the Landes family did. They simply told the cancer specialist Alice wanted to go home, and that meant a hospice referral. It also meant the siblings would have to pull together and get past long-standing resentments to give Alice the loving, calm care she needed and deserved. They hoped hospice would keep her comfortable. They had no idea how much it would help them to put aside old hurts, reach a fragile peace, and be there for both their parents and for one another. Years later, Jeanne would observe, "The end of life is like an earthquake. You just don't prepare."

As it happened, the cascade of events began with a different natural disaster. On a business trip in Miami, Jeanne had called her parents to let them know she was trying to get a flight home before a major hurricane came ashore. At forty-two, Jeanne always checked in with her parents when she traveled because she knew they worried. This time she picked up something strange in her mother's voice. She thought she had a bad connection or Alice was nervous about her safety.

Just to be sure, another sister, Barbara, took Alice to her primary care doctor. A chest X-ray showed a lump in her breast, which at first seemed like good news — a lump could be removed, they thought — but the doctor sent Alice to the local hospital immediately for more definitive tests. There she had more lab work, a breast biopsy, MRI's, head and body scans. Salinas Valley Memorial Hospital, on the Central Coast of California, kept Alice overnight. When Jeanne arrived the next morning, she found her frightened mother alone and disoriented, held to the bed by soft restraints.

Alice, an immigrant from China, had learned English as an adult, but, whatever had been explained to her in the hospital, she didn't understand why she was there. Jeanne spoke to her mother in Chinese and learned that Alice had gotten up during the night to use the restroom and slipped. To keep her from falling again, she was tethered to the bed. Jeanne had the restraints removed.

A young oncologist explained that Alice had lung cancer that had spread to her brain, which was why she had difficulty speaking. What Jeanne had noticed as "something different" about her speech turned out to be seizures brought on by brain swelling. The one bit of good news brought little solace — the breast lump was benign.

The oncologist had scheduled a bone marrow biopsy, which would take about half an hour and require sedation. They already knew the cancer had metastasized not only to Alice's brain but also her bones, beyond hope for a cure. The doctor said she might live four months.

Jeanne translated for her mother.

"If that is the case, then that is the case," her mother responded in Chinese.

"What do you want to do?" Jeanne asked.

"I want to go home."

The siblings struggled to accept her decision, telling their father not to worry about the house; nobody planned to sell it anytime soon. Alice kept repeating her wish. Jeanne told the doctor to cancel the bone marrow procedure. "We don't need to know any more."

They left the hospital with medications for Alice's low-grade fever and seizures, twenty-four-hour numbers to call the hospice for help, and *Gone from My Sight* ("The Hospice Blue Book"), by Barbara Karnes, a hospice nurse. It was set up much the way child development books offer tips for different stages. As with growing children, no dying patient follows the book page by page. But for caregivers and patients, just as for new parents, knowing what might happen and when to call the doctor is a great help. The Wuns also received a kit of pain medication, just in case.

A Houseful of Strangers

Ying and Alice (born Oi Quehn) Wun were married as teenagers in Guangzhou (Canton), in 1937. He had come to this country just before World War II, served in the Army, and in 1947 went back to China to bring his wife to Salinas. With the help of an affluent benefactor and the GI Bill, Ying opened the United Café at 1 Main Street. Today that is the site of the National Steinbeck Center, highlighting the literature of new immigrants like the Wuns. It is named for Nobel Prize-winning (and Salinas-born) author John Steinbeck, whose most famous book, *The Grapes of Wrath,* tracked a poor family of farmers moving from the Oklahoma Dust Bowl to California in search of a better life.

Alice worked in the café until they sold it in 1985. She never smoked, and, although many people in the café did, her cancer, adenocarcinoma, often afflicts non-smokers. It is the most common lung cancer found in women and the most common among all Asians. As in Alice's case, it may be present for many years before causing any symptoms and go undiagnosed until it is far advanced.

When Ying arrived home from the hospital, he found strangers busying themselves in his house — lots of strangers, because in their first experience with hospice the Wun siblings welcomed all the varieties of help on offer. The sisters had cleaned out a room so that Salinas Hospice, a small nonprofit, could bring in a hospital bed and an oxygen tank. Ying panicked. Suddenly he was on the edge of losing his wife of fifty-four years, and all these people occupied his home. He felt he did not belong. Nor was he about to discuss his feelings, or anyone else's. He told Jeanne he just had to leave.

At seventy, Ying did not drive, he was distraught, and he had no plan. So while the other sisters settled their mother into the hospital bed and new schedule, Jeanne drove their father to a friend's house an hour away. Maybe he would settle down after a few days. But they got to Santa Cruz late in the evening, and Ying did not want to stay. He felt he didn't belong there either. Jeanne drove him to her house in San Jose, another forty-five minute trip, and within the week they returned to Salinas.

A hospice home health aide showed the sisters how to bathe and change Alice and rotate her in bed. Barbara took over the cooking. She had always been angry with her father for forcing her to work at the restaurant as a child, but she had learned her way around a kitchen.

At times when their mother refused to eat, they were frantic. What had they done wrong? They were failing. They called the hospice nurse, who explained that someone so sick didn't always need to eat. They had grown up hearing that a dying elder must have food in her stomach, or she could be fated to wander the mythical "realm of hungry ghosts." The nurse helped them to see their mother's refusal to eat as a natural process of death, not a bad reflection on their filial devotion.

Similarly, the nurse assured them that it was natural and they were not to blame when Alice pulled the oxygen tubes out of her nose. She needed to feel she had some control over her life. The message to the family was not a rebuke or a desperate scream of "Leave me alone I just want to die." It was a sensible choice under the circumstances, a statement that "I don't need this now." And she didn't. She was breathing on her own.

As promised, the four daughters upended their lives to care for their mother. Virginia, who lived in Seattle, got a leave of absence from Microsoft and took the first two months as primary caregiver. Then Nancy Chin, the youngest sister, came from Southern California for a month. In San Jose, Jeanne's employer, Quantum, a disk storage manufacturer, allowed her to go part-time and work remotely. She often stayed overnight in Salinas to give Virginia a break. Barbara cut back to three days a week on her job at the Salinas Post Office and spent the rest of her time at the house. It felt odd to be together there again, and odder still to think about how they hadn't been together in so long, considering how close they had once been.

The Wuns' seven children all were born about a year apart. Except for their father's sister in San Jose, they had no extended family in the United States. They were it for each other. They played cowboys and Indians in their own house, not with the neighborhood kids.

During the first month on hospice, Alice could walk with assistance and was able to leave the house as long as she had her anti-seizure medications. One day, the four sisters drove her to Monterey, where she used to love to walk along the wharf. Other days, grandchildren visited.

With help from hospice, siblings who had spun into independent orbits wobbled tentatively back into the one they once shared. Barbara videotaped the trees and flowers around the house, so Alice could see familiar sights when she could no longer go outside.

But as weary days and nights blended into another, Jeanne and her siblings felt over-whelmed and uncertain, testy and unap-preciated. They fretted about every move they made to help their mother, and whether they were helping her at all.

A hospice social worker came and listened to everyone's concerns, including Ying's, re-assuring them they were all doing the best they could. The social worker came back several times to speak privately with Ying.

They also accepted the offer of a hospice volunteer to visit and the suggestion to keep a journal of their mother's care, to literally get them all on the same page.

October 6 journal entry by Virginia: Decided to start beefing up Mom's meals to three meals and grazing in between . . . small por-tions and alternating with ice chips. Mom is a shaker and a mover in bed during the night. . . . Has a sense of humor and laughs when we tell her stories.

October 8 journal entry by Virginia: [Mom] escaped to San Jose. Mom's idea. Took three of us to make this work. Used Barbara's car. Jeanne brought home some Chinese goodies and fresh tofu for Mom.

October 9 journal entry by Jeanne: A good day. Played mah jongg for four hours. [Mom] sat in favorite chair. 730p [Mom] rang bell for BM [bowel movement]! Yeah! Urine: 39.5.

The Estranged Son

When Jeanne asked her mother if there was anyone she wanted to see, she knew the answer before Alice opened her mouth: "Gene." The second-oldest son had been estranged from the family for twenty years. While the oldest brother, Sonny, had been quick-tempered, Gene had been dependable, kind, often the favorite of his parents and others. When Barbara was little, she would wake him up to take her to the bathroom at night. Later he was the one to help with her homework. He kept them all together as a family when they started going their own ways as teenagers.

Gene had married into another Chinese family in Salinas, and there had been a deep rift during the prenuptial planning. Nobody had seen Gene in years. He lived in Sacramento, more than three hours away. His sons were strangers to their paternal grandparents, uncles, and aunts. They felt they had lost a brother, and a central thread in their family.

Jeanne called and told Gene, "Mom is sick; she would like to see you." He came alone on a Greyhound bus, afraid he would be too upset to make the long drive.

All the siblings were at the house that day. They accepted ground rules that this visit was for Mom, that if there were arguments they'd take them outside. Gene arrived and greetings were superficial but cordial. Jeanne brought him in to see his mother, and turned off the baby monitor so they would have privacy. Alice was obviously pleased to see him after all these years. But when he emerged, he got an earful, the buildup of two decades of a beloved brother's disappearance. Ying just listened, and packed Gene a lunch for the bus ride back.

In her third month of hospice, Alice slept more. She might nod or move her head from side to side, but she rarely spoke, and then only in Chinese. She sometimes looked off, toward something no one else could see, as if taking a little visit beyond this life. The hospice nurse assured them that this too was normal.

The young oncologist who had referred them to hospice kept in touch by phone. In the fourth month, she called to say she wanted to visit. Alice clearly remembered the doctor and brightened so much to see her that Jeanne said, "Gosh, we might have another week or more!"

The doctor nodded and said gently, "It's near."

That evening and into the next day, Alice slept more deeply again. But they continued talking to her and told her that Nancy was on her way. She left her house at six o'clock in the morning and ran into heavy rain that broke her windshield wipers. Nancy found a public phone to tell her sisters where she was, but then the car wouldn't start. She prayed. It turned over, and she didn't stop again. About fifteen minutes after Nancy came through the door, Alice died, surrounded by three daughters and her husband.

The sisters bathed and clothed her, and, as in Chinese tradition, Ying placed a couple of symbolic items in her hands, to signify that they were parting ways in this life. Because she had died at home and not in an ICU, the family was able to leave her body in bed through the next morning, so that all the siblings would have a chance to get there and say goodbye.

Alice wanted no funeral, just cremation and her ashes scattered at sea. A friend with a small boat in Monterey Bay could take five passengers: the three sisters, Ying, and Gene. The rest of the family met them later at a nearby Chinese restaurant. Their mother's final months had brought them together again, at least around this table.

The Widower

Ying Wun's younger sister came to live with him. Auntie, as everyone in the family called her, took over the household and prepared Chinese herbal medicines and soups, and the widower gradually returned to old routines. If he went anywhere, it was to the cardiologist monitoring his enlarged heart.

Jeanne, however, did not bounce back. She sobbed every night on the drive home from work. The family tradition was not to talk about death, but she had to find an outlet. She opened the phone book and found Hospice of the Valley, ten minutes from her house.

Jeanne met a couple of times with a bereavement counselor, who helped her see that she wasn't losing her mind, and she joined a group for people who had lost parents. She stayed through the first anniversary of her mother's death, and it helped so much that she volunteered to work in grief care. Soon she found herself on the nonprofit's board of directors, with a new sense of purpose. When Hospice of the Valley offered her a job, Jeanne jumped at the opportunity.

Eventually, Ying's heart condition worsened, and his cardiologist suggested his quality of life would improve if he had surgery to install a pacemaker. It would help his heart beat at a better rhythm and give him more energy.

Jeanne was shocked when he told the doctor: "Why would I want to live longer than what is natural for me?"

In the past, her father might have embraced whatever medical technology was offered. But since being hospitalized with painful kidney stones, he was done with surgeries and hospitals. The pacemaker also would raise another end-of-life issue for the family: Once installed, the device would not stop by itself. Someone would have to make the decision to turn it off.

Again, Ying was clear: "I came in with this one, I'll leave with this one." All he wanted to know now was that he didn't have cancer, the disease that had killed his wife, and the doctor assured him that was so.

"And you don't have to come here anymore," the doctor said. "A nurse will come to your house." Her father was happy, while Jeanne left the doctor's office in tears.

They hadn't mentioned the word *hospice*, but when Jeanne had said, "Don't worry, Dad, we'll take care of you, just like we took care of Mom," he knew what she meant. And now he wanted to get out, just as Alice had. He, Auntie, Jeanne, and Barbara took a day trip to Monterey. They took roses from his yard and threw them into the water to be with Alice.

In January 2007, Ying allowed hospice to install a hospital bed in his room, to make caregiving easier on his daughters. This was a tactic they had learned from hospice with their mother: frame it as their parent taking care of them.

Gene visited again, and one day toward the end he fed his father with a spoon. He told Barbara he would take time off from work to come and help, but that weekend, Easter Sunday 2007, Ying died peacefully, of heart failure. He was eighty-six.

Again, the whole family gathered at a Chinese restaurant. In hopes of a continued reconciliation, Barbara gave a white chocolate dove to each sibling.

Jeanne, Barbara, and Nancy still see each other a lot. Nancy and Virginia instant-message each other. The surviving family connection is the Salinas house, empty for three years since Auntie moved in with Jeanne. They hadn't gotten around to putting it up for sale.

CHAPTER SIX:
PETER SERRELL: FINAL FAST

"We don't have a choice about whether we're going to die, but sometimes we have a choice about whether that's going to be easier or harder."

A few weeks before his ninety-fourth birthday, Peter Serrell was hospitalized for severe gut pain. Tests found nothing definitive and after a few days he seemed to improve. His doctor suspected colitis and told him to try eating and see how he felt. But Peter had a different idea. He called his oldest daughter, Barbara Serrell Hansen, to take him home. He would stop eating and drinking until he died.

This happens more commonly than most of us realize. People facing the end of their lives who do not want to let things drag out may move them along fairly simply, and legally, by fasting, as long as they are capable of making the decision. Hospices often provide comfort and family support — essentially, doing what hospice is supposed to do for any patient with a terminal condition and a life expectancy of six months or less.

Peter had talked before about fasting to death. He had osteoporosis and heart pains. His legs had become so weak he could barely get around, even with a rolling walker. His back hurt constantly from two spinal fractures in the past decade. His teeth were weakening, and the dentist recommended extraction and dentures. Meanwhile, he had to live on soups and purees like a toddler. It was relentless decline punctuated by the occasional medical crisis, which of course never happened on a Tuesday afternoon but in the middle of the night. He had to wake up his wife and Barbara, his only local daughter, who lived across town.

Although he always pulled through, each emergency knocked him a little further downhill. Nothing Peter ever said suggested that he wanted to die, but he accepted that he would. He hated the prospect of losing his independence or spending his last days gazing helplessly over the rails of a hospital bed.

The first time Peter brought up the idea

of fasting was in the summer of 2008. His three daughters calmly heard him out. This was not a family to plead and sob to get their way or to duck the subject of dying. Peter's youngest daughter, Elizabeth Menkin — Betty, to her family and friends — was a hospice physician in California. One of Betty's three daughters, Nora, worked as a funeral director in Seattle. Peter's wife of sixty-three years, Kathleen, had died in 2003, after she stopped taking her heart medication when she learned she had Alzheimer's. She spent her final weeks happily dining on bacon and other artery-clogging favorites. "It's been sort of a family understanding that if you wanted to check out, you could turn your head to the wall and say, 'I'm leaving now,' " said Peter's middle daughter, Beverly Serrell.

But in the summer of 2008 nobody was ready for Peter to leave, not his daughters or his new wife, Becky Koch, or, in hindsight, Peter himself. His daughters listed all sorts of reasons why he should hang in, and it would become family lore that what finally persuaded him was this: if he died, he would not be able to vote for Barack Obama for president.

Peter mentioned fasting again a few days after the election, and his doctor put him on the antidepressant Wellbutrin. It accomplished nothing — Peter was not depressed. But he could not resist Becky's good home cooking, and the idea seemed to fade.

"This time I mean it," Peter told Barbara when he left the hospital in late 2008. As she drove him home through the streets of Portland, Oregon, she wondered what had sealed the decision. Was this latest emergency the last straw? Did the empty hours in the hospital remind him how much he did not want to die there? Did the quick Alzheimer's test in the hospital scare him into taking control while he could? The doctor had tossed out three random words — simple ones, like fish, pencil, and daffodil. Ten minutes later, he asked Peter to repeat them back.

"Gulp," Peter said. "I don't remember."

In the car, Barbara did not question Peter about his decision. She simply acknowledged his resolve. "I am so sorry to hear it," she told him. He said he knew that his act would be hard on the family, but he needed them to let him go ahead. And they did.

Taking Control

"We don't have a choice about whether we're going to die, but sometimes we have a choice about whether that's going to be easier or harder," Betty Menkin said. No hospice would encourage a decision like Peter's, but any decent one would be there to help. Nobody would call the act suicide, a word loaded with implications of irrational behavior, desperation, even cowardice and sin. A patient who wants to fast to death does not have to stockpile pills or ask a family member to commit a crime, however well intentioned, by administering a deadly dose of morphine. Nor does the patient have to move to the Netherlands or to one of the three states — Oregon, Washington, and Vermont — that allow doctors to prescribe lethal medication for competent, terminal patients. (Montana could be considered the fourth, but the law is less specific. The state Supreme Court ruled in 2009 that Montana's living will law protects doctors from prosecution for writing such prescriptions. Since then, several state legislators have introduced bills both to permit and regulate physician-assisted suicide, and to outlaw it, but none of the measures has gone anywhere.)

Law books do not say much about fasting, but they make clear that a competent patient has the right to forego life-saving treatments, from ventilators, kidney dialysis, and chemotherapy to run-of-the-mill antibiotics. Many ethicists and hospices view food and water in the same light. It's your body. You get to choose what goes in.

It is impossible to say how often sick people consciously refuse food and water to speed up dying, and rely on hospices for help. The only published study on the question surveyed 307 hospice nurses in Oregon, and 126 of them, or 41 percent, said that at some point they'd had at least one patient who decided to fast to death. In almost all cases, the patient followed through. It's a small sample, skewed by geography. Oregon, where Peter happened to live, takes a kinder view of these things than do most places in America. More people there sign advance care directives and use hospices than in the nation as a whole. It was the first state to legalize physician-assisted suicide, a practice that runs counter to the hospice philosophy. (A recent study found that 85 percent to 95 percent of people in Oregon and Washington who choose legal assisted suicide also use hospice services. This leaves workers struggling to honor the principles of compassion and non-abandonment without violating the hospice code of allowing death to occur naturally yet doing nothing to hasten it. Seventy-five percent of hospice organizations do not permit workers to be present when a fatal dose of medication is used.)

Fasting does not have the legal and ethical baggage of assisted suicide or euthanasia — for a few reasons. First, the patient controls every step. Nobody else has to write a special prescription, turn up the dial on the drug pump, or do anything to hasten dying. Second, it takes about ten days to two weeks to die, so the deed is not impulsive. Peter remained clear-headed for a week after he stopped eating and drinking. He sometimes sat with his family during meals. He had time to change his mind.

Third, many patients naturally lose their appetite at the very end of life and stop eating without a big announcement. While Peter asserted his wishes, his daughters would later suspect that he had simply been giving voice to a biological imperative that even he did not recognize — his body was shutting down and did not need food any more than a car without an engine needs gas. Betty had seen many hospice and nursing home patients nibble food or sip juice only because relatives nagged and begged them to do so. "It gets to the point where we tell families: he's not dying because he's not eating — he's not eating because he's dying," she said.

For those of us who cannot make it from breakfast to lunch without a growling stomach, it can be hard to imagine that fasting is a relatively painless, peaceful way to die. Starvation conjures images of horrific suffering — the piles of skeletal victims in Nazi death camps, the distended bellies of babies in Darfur. Peter would die not of starvation but of dehydration, and the difference is not mere semantics. Starvation — eating less food than the body burns up, while continuing to drink fluids — slowly shrinks muscles, including the heart. People grow thinner and thinner until they no longer have the strength to breathe. It happens over agonizing months. Dehydration does not rob muscle and flesh but changes the blood chemistry, fatally, over a week or two. Rising sodium levels can cause drowsiness and put a patient into a coma near the end. The spike in potassium can cause heart problems. Without water to eliminate waste, the kidneys fail.

When Peter returned home from the hospital, he told Becky of his decision and called his other two daughters. Betty flew to Portland the next day and got Peter enrolled in a local hospice program. He fit the criteria of "debility unspecified" — a hospice category for frail old people who have a long list of medical problems and a short life expectancy if they no longer pursue treatment, but who have no clear-cut terminal illness such as pancreatic cancer. ("Death by a thousand paper cuts," is how the Hospice Doctor blog describes it.)

In some ways, the hospice experience would disappoint Peter's family, Betty most of all. The first nurse on the scene spent an hour filling out forms, asking what everyone in the family considered "cover-your-ass questions." She never did what Betty considered the first rule of hospice care: get to know the patient and the family and understand their "goals of care" — what do they want out of the time that's left? It rankled Peter's wife, Becky, that the nurse assumed she was his housekeeper.

A visit from a hospice social worker a few days later went better — she spent time talking with Peter. But nobody in the family would feel much connection with the hospice team. It was sadly ironic, given that one family member had devoted nearly a quarter of a century to providing hospice care and championing the hospice cause. Then again, Betty readily attended to the few problems that came up, so the family did not ask for much from the hospice. For example, at three o'clock one morning, she put on Latex gloves and cleaned Peter's bowel because he was constipated. Another family would have phoned the hospice for help, and a nurse probably would have driven right over. An emergency visit in the middle of the night from a competent, compassionate hospice professional might have overshadowed and even erased the family's initial irritation with the bureaucracy.

Even though the hospice service fell short, Betty did not regret signing her father up. By accepting and supporting Peter's decision to fast, the hospice made it seem as OK, as normal, as any other way of dying. "Hospice provided permission," Betty said.

Not that Peter needed it.

The Sacred Act of Caring

Peter was a fixer — faulty engines, broken appliances, shattered hearts. As a young mechanical engineer in the 1940s, he worked at the new Jet Propulsion Laboratory in Pasadena, California, helping to build wind tunnels for testing the world's first rockets. Nearly a half-century later, after his forty-seven-year-old daughter, Elaine, was killed in a head-on crash with a young woman drunk on peppermint schnapps, Peter initiated a reconciliation

151

process with the driver. Others in the family resisted at first. Who wanted to sit in a room with that monster? But eventually they went along, warily, and Peter's instincts proved right. The fury and crushing grief they all had felt began to lift after they came face-to-face with the young woman, said what they had to say, and heard her sincere regret and desire to make amends. Elaine's husband later wrote in his journal that he felt renewed.

Until his early eighties, Peter picked up his oars every morning, climbed on a bus, and rode to the shore of the Willamette River for an hour of sculling. That's where he fractured his spine the first time. He'd been stepping out of the scull when it jerked in the wake of a powerboat, knocking him on his butt. It laid him up for three months. He relished telling people that he was the only one in his old folks home to have a sports injury, and, although someone could quibble with this description of his vibrant senior living community, his claim was probably true. Only later would he realize that the accident triggered his decline. He had to give up sculling but found less physically demanding ways to stay active.

Every week he reserved a library book or two online and rode the bus and tram downtown to pick up his reading and return the previous week's books. Then he took the bus home, making sure to board within a two-hour window so he could complete the round trip on a one-dollar senior-fare ticket. An avowed agnostic, he regularly attended a Unitarian church, where he was the oldest member, by far, of a men's fellowship that had been meeting for twenty-five years. "He believed in community more than he believed in God," Betty said. "Taking care of other people was sacred."

Peter had ninety people at his ninetieth birthday party. Two years later he married one of them, Becky Koch, a 79-year-old neighbor he had gotten to know while they shot pool in the clubroom of their complex. They threw a reception for the whole place, 175 people. They ordered 800 pieces of sushi, and, in a sly nod to their cue-stick courtship, they covered the cocktail tables with cloths of billiard-green.

Peter suffered his second spinal fracture when he fell in the shower. This recovery took even longer than the first and left him frailer than ever. He was shrinking too, because of osteoporosis, especially in his torso, and became stooped. He still dressed every morning in his trademark outfit — khaki pants, long-sleeved plaid shirt, dark socks, and sandals. But he no longer felt secure enough on his feet to leave the building, and he had fewer and fewer places he cared to go. His teeth problems made eating a chore, which killed the fun of going out for sushi. He stopped going to the library, because, he told Betty, he had finished every book he wanted to read.

Around that time, Betty was developing a deck of cards to give people a simple way to figure out what kind of end-of-life care they wanted. She called it Go Wish, a play on that childhood favorite, Go Fish. The cards describe experiences that, according to research, people value as death approaches — for instance, "to be free of pain" or "to die at home." The idea is to sort through thirty-six cards and prioritize ten. A "wild card" lets you write a wish if you did not find it in the deck. Peter served as a beta tester and wrote down his top ten wishes. Betty would later reproduce the list in an essay in the *Journal of Palliative Medicine.*

His number one wish, his wild card, was "to be offered adult food that I can accept or reject." Peter said he also hoped to experience human touch, remember personal accomplishments, have someone who would listen to him, and maintain his dignity.

Becky stashed the paper in a drawer. It would become a kind of operating manual for his final days.

Feasting on Life

Peter started his fast on a Monday, and the apartment was packed for the rest of the week. Neighbors and men from his church fellowship came. Two granddaughters flew in, and he Skyped with the third. Beverly arrived Friday from Chicago.

Every morning Peter dressed as usual, from plaid shirt to khakis to socks and sandals. He sat in the living room with his family, looking at faded photos in aging, bulky albums. He told stories of his youth, of growing up as the only child of older parents and of riding a horse in what were then the wilds of Southern California to the beach. He talked about his work and, for the first time, his daughters appreciated what it meant to engineer a wind tunnel in a pre-digital era, using mechanical pencils, paper, and a head for math. The daughters told stories too — how Peter used to squeeze fresh orange juice and make buckwheat pancakes for Sunday breakfast, and how they confided in him, not their mother, because he listened better and did not criticize. Betty later described these days in her essay in the *Journal of Palliative Medicine:* "Instead of drinking water, he drank from the well-springs of connections with friends and family."

If Peter felt stomach pangs or a hunger headache, he showed no signs and said nothing. The only apparent discomfort that first week was dry mouth. He used special swabs and brushed his teeth for relief. He joined his family at dinner one evening in the dining room of the complex, taking part in the conversation while ignoring the food. One night, he accepted a lick of chocolate ice cream and then said "no, thanks" to more.

Becky answered the phone one day, and the daughter of an acquaintance lashed out, practically shouting that Peter's family was guilty of elder abuse. Becky stood, speechless. Betty took the receiver, listened for a few seconds, told the caller to mind her business, and hung up.

"Ah," Peter said, with a dismissive wave of the hand, "She's crazy."

On day seven of the fast, just before Betty left for the airport to return to work, she thought back to Peter's Go Wish list and his desire for human touch. She lay down alongside him in his queen-size bed. Her daughter stretched out on his other side. They called it "a girl sandwich" and huddled close.

That day and the next, Peter got dressed in the morning but stayed mostly in bed. Fewer visitors came, and he seemed content to listen to conversations without saying much. When Beverly found herself alone with her dad, she asked him a question she had long wondered about but had never felt comfortable broaching: Did he regret that he'd never had a son?

No, he said. He'd been small, geeky, a misfit as a child. He never particularly wanted to raise boys because he thought they might remind him of his early unhappiness.

Peter slept through most of day nine. Beverly watched him breathe in and out, in and out, and then stop — was he dead? Then his breathing resumed. "It was like watching the ocean pulling away and then come back, pulling away and then come back," she said later.

He was agitated that night and, for the first time, not entirely lucid. He kept trying to get out of bed to go to the bathroom. Becky put on a diaper, but he worried about soiling the bed. He moaned a bit, and Becky and Beverly feared he was in pain. They gave him some of the drugs the hospice nurse had left — morphine drops under the tongue and anti-anxiety medicine. He fell asleep, and Becky slid into bed beside him.

When she woke up in the morning, Peter was lying on his back with his eyes closed and his left arm bent at the elbow. She walked into the living room, where Beverly slept on the sofa. Becky gently nudged Beverly and said Peter was dead.

For a long time afterward, Beverly questioned her decision to give him morphine. She knew it did not kill him at that small dose. But it troubled her to think that it may have put him in a place he did not want to be, somewhere he could not feel the comfort of her hand stroking his arm or the warmth of Becky's body beside his.

Her sisters had no qualms about Peter's last night. Sure, they cried and missed him. But they imagined him somewhere doing a Rocky Balboa victory dance, with arms outstretched and fists pumping the air. In the months that followed, Betty saw many patients who made her recall with gratitude that her father had lived and died exactly as he wanted, sometimes because her patients did too and she could see how much it meant to them and their families, and sometimes because her patients did not.

At Peter's memorial service, everyone in the family paid tribute to his grit and independence in a way he would have loved. They all came dressed in khakis, plaid shirts, socks, and sandals.

Chapter Seven:
Fred Holliday: Inside the Catch-22 of Hospice

"Dying isn't hard. Getting paid by Medicare is."

The Washington Home and Community Hospices, on a leafy street in the tony Upper Northwest corridor of the nation's capital, is four miles from the White House. Five successive presidents, from Jimmy Carter to George W. Bush, have come on official visits, paying homage to the work done here. Princess Diana paid a call on her first official visit to the United States, a trip that stirred such a royal tizzy that crowds had to be kept from blocking traffic in the city. She stayed forty minutes, visiting about forty patients on the nursing-home side of the building and all four patients in the hospice wing. She held the hand of a man with throat cancer who doctors feared might die just before she arrived. He could not talk but he looked up at her and formed a circle with his thumb and index finger, the OK sign.

The home has also logged many Washington notables as patients, once-mighty lawyers and writers, Pentagon brass, a CIA field agent or two. But the best-known person to come here to die was the syndicated newspaper columnist Art Buchwald, the most widely read political satirist of his day. The cigar-chomping Pulitzer Prize–winner spent decades chronicling the foibles and hypocrisies of the power elite, with delight and homespun wit. He covered even more presidents than have visited the Washington Home — nine, going back to Kennedy. In one of the last pieces Buchwald ever wrote, he turned his eye for the absurd toward the system that regulates and pays for hospice. "Dying isn't hard," he wrote. "Getting paid by Medicare is."

The story of how Buchwald learned this began in the fall of 2005, just before his eightieth birthday. He had his right leg amputated below the knee because of a dangerous blockage in an artery, and he started dialysis because his kidneys were failing. He hated being tethered to a machine three times a week for five hours at a stretch. After twelve treatments, he refused to continue. He entered the hospice in early

February 2006. His doctor said that, without a machine doing the job of his kidneys and cleansing his blood of waste and toxins, Buchwald would die before the end of the month.

Except that he didn't. Inexplicably, his kidneys started working. Through the window of his private room — all the rooms in the hospice unit are private and have large windows overlooking gardens with flagstone paths, wrought iron tables and chairs, fountains, and a turtle pond — Buchwald could see first the President's Day storm that dumped ten inches of snow, then the first buds of the trees turning to full flower, and finally the flowers giving way to the green canopy of late spring. In the hospice sitting room, where efforts have been made, more or less successfully, to mask the institutional look with a homier aesthetic — twin tweed couches, twin taupe wingback chairs, dark wooden tables, a library, and a big-screen TV — Buchwald entertained a parade of celebrity friends, including a few Kennedys.

"Washington's Hottest Salon is a Deathbed," a *New York Times* headline announced. Visitors brought food, and Buchwald devoured blintzes, cheesecake, and other favorites he had given up long before

162

in the name of health. He wrote his column, planned his funeral, and gave media interviews about his odd predicament as "the man who wouldn't die."

After a few weeks in the hospice, Medicare would no longer cover his stay. The program generally pays for inpatient hospice care until patients are stable enough to go home, and most private insurance plans follow that formula. Saying he was having "a swell time" in the hospice, "the best time of my life," Buchwald paid to stay put and penned a book about the experience, *Too Soon to Say Goodbye.*

In July, he felt strong enough to go to his home on Martha's Vineyard, his summertime haunt for forty-five years. He returned to Washington in September and showed up on the party circuit to celebrate the publication of his book in late fall. He died in his son's house in January 2007.

From Death's Door Back to Life

Fred Holliday is a more typical example of what happens when the rules say it's time for a patient to go home from a hospice. Fred was thirty-nine. He had kidney cancer that had spread to his lungs, spine, hips, pelvis, and femur, turning bones so brittle they could snap like twigs. From the time he'd been diagnosed, just two-and-a-half months earlier, he had been moved from one facility to another — forty-five transports in all. His wife, Regina, kept count.

She thought the transport to the inpatient hospice at Washington Home, on the night of May 20, 2009, would be his last. So did the emergency medical technicians in the ambulance. They had transported Fred before, and they liked him — how could you not like a film studies professor who had written his doctoral dissertation about *Buffy the Vampire Slayer*, which he insisted dealt with death better than any other show on television? They had gotten to know Regina too. She always rode along, and though she sat up front, next to the driver, Fred felt her calming presence and relaxed.

In a strange way, he had come to look forward to ambulance rides. The jostling of a gurney hurt like hell and could be dangerous — during a bed-to-gurney transfer when he first entered the hospital, an orderly had carelessly shoved his hip, cracking it. But these rides got Fred outdoors for a few minutes, the only time that happened anymore. It usually lifted his spirits to smell air washed clean by rain, feel the breeze on his face, or look up and see sky instead of the pallid acoustical tile of a hospital.

On the way to the hospice, the techs tried talking with Fred, but he was lethargic and fading. Regina, usually a rock, started crying. One of the techs cried quietly too. As Fred was whisked inside, the techs wondered if he would make it through the night.

The next morning, he was sitting up in bed and spooning down applesauce, the first food he had eaten in days. His cheeks had color, and he asked Regina to bring their sons, Isaac, then three years old, and Freddie, age ten, to see him. The reversal seemed miraculous to Regina, but it was just good palliative medicine. Like the people in the before-and-after slides Cicely Saunders used to display during her lectures, patients can come into hospice seemingly on the brink of death and once their pain, nausea, or delirium are effectively controlled, they rally. It happens so often that it has a name: the hospice spurt. The phenomenon seems counterintuitive, especially if you think of hospice as "giving up." Until that morning, Regina did.

She and Fred did not choose hospice — not in the Buchwald sense, at least. If any of the doctors Fred had seen during his ordeal had proposed a treatment to extend his life, the Hollidays would have grabbed it, no matter how brutal the side effects. Then again, in hindsight Regina would say that if a doctor had told them honestly that his cancer was too far advanced for any therapy or surgery to change its course, that to try simply for the sake of trying would probably do nothing but compound his suffering, the couple might have opted for hospice sooner. But neither conversation took place.

Instead, Fred had been transferred from one hospital to another, from the second hospital to a rehabilitation center, from rehab to a third hospital, while a succession of doctors tried to pull him out of the latest crisis, sometimes caused not by his illness but by the care he received. In hospital number two, he underwent surgery to pin the hip that was broken but never diagnosed in hospital number one. After the operation, he was sent to rehab to relearn to walk before undergoing any cancer surgery, even though Regina told the doctors that Fred had stopped walking before the fracture because he was so weak. The medical team at the rehab center switched his painkillers, leaving him in constant agony on top of incontinence, exhaustion, and anemia. Regina demanded a blood transfusion — he had received them in the first two hospitals, and they had fortified him. So one night Fred was wheeled into an ambulance and driven to the nearest hospital, across the parking lot. Insurance rules required a vehicle transport.

The transfusion perked him up. The doctor on duty reviewed his history with more attention and kindness than any other physician had shown, and wondered why on earth she would send a man with stage 4 renal-cell carcinoma back to rehab for physical therapy. She asked Regina if they had considered hospice.

By morning the doctor was off duty, leaving Regina alone to enter Fred's room, sit down on his bed, and bring up the topic.

"Hospice?" he said. "I'm going to die?"

She cried and said she was so sorry. She told him he would be able to spend time with the kids.

"OK, Reggie, if that's what you think is best."

She did not know what to think. It felt like life in freefall, as if she and Fred had tumbled down a hole, rolling and shouting futilely for help until they now hit bottom hard. But, once Fred got settled in Washington Home, it did seem best — near paradise compared with every other stop along this awful journey. The night he came in, the hospice physician put him back on his original painkiller, Dilaudid, and a steroid, and his pain ebbed. The staff looked Fred in the eye, which made a big impression on both him and Regina, after months in hospitals where everyone avoided his gaze, as if his illness were shameful.

The hospice facility, so welcoming to Art Buchwald's well-connected friends, beautifully accommodated a young family in distress. The boys could hang out in the sitting room, watch television, and play in the gardens. This helped Freddie, especially, who had autism. The noise, odors, and frenzy of the hospitals had been torture for him. He had withdrawn from everyone, his father most of all. But he did not mind the hospice. It was quiet. It smelled fine. He could bring his dad McDonald's burgers and shakes and watch them disappear off the grease-soaked paper. When Freddie got agitated, Regina took him to play by the turtle pond. She hoped it brought him solace. At least it distracted him.

The hospice was not perfect. It had no WiFi, so Regina could not post on Facebook or lotsahelpinghands.com, her lifelines since the nightmare had begun. The hospice worried about computer security and most patients were much older and did not seem to care. But Regina relied on social media to send out last-minute calls for a babysitter, invite friends to visit on Fred's good days, ask them to stay away on bad days, and simply stay in touch with the living world.

Fred did not like the hospice food. "Other than that," Regina said, "he loved it."

Take Two Pills and Call Me in the Morning

Fred Holliday and Regina McCanless met in an art class at Oklahoma State University in 1992. She was a sophomore, five-foot one-inch tall, with thick, long red hair. He was a graduate student in film studies and towered over her by ten inches. He told her he fell in love standing behind her, watching her paint. They married the following year.

A dozen years later, they were living in Washington, raising their sons and juggling about a half-dozen part-time jobs. Fred taught college-level film courses. Regina taught art to preschoolers and managed the art department in a toy store. They lived in a one-bedroom apartment, and they had no health insurance. Fred suffered occasional pain from a urethra stricture, a narrowing of the urinary tube, but he knew the family could not afford the $20,000 surgery, and he postponed treatment.

Their fortunes lifted in late summer of 2008. Fred secured a one-year appointment at American University, a dream opportunity. He loved the job. He ate lunch in the department lounge rather than in his cramped office and talked with everyone who wandered through. He quickly made a few friends among the faculty, who found him refreshing — a brilliant scholar without a shred of pretention. Fred knew his critical theory, and he could expound at length on esoteric Chinese cinema, but he showed as much enthusiasm for Stephen King, Harry Potter, and zombie flicks. Best of all, he was not embarrassed about it. He inspired several colleagues to read *The Dark Tower* and watch *Dawn of the Dead.*

In January 2009, Fred felt a stabbing pain in his rib. Now with health insurance through the university, he went to an internist. An X-ray revealed a fracture, which seemed weird because he had not fallen recently or taken a punch. But the family had passed around a winter cold and respiratory tract infection, and the doctor said he probably cracked his rib coughing. She sent him home with a prescription for a painkiller.

Then the pain shifted to his back, somewhere deep, and worsened. It felt as if someone had drilled nails into his lower spine. The doctor prescribed a stronger painkiller, which helped no more than the first. He lost weight, had night sweats, and became anemic, but dragged himself to work and put on a good front. No one there knew anything was wrong until one day in March, when a colleague, Michael Wenthe, found him in the parking lot, too sick to walk to class. Fred asked Michael to drive him home.

Fred returned to the doctor, who asked him if he was depressed. No, he said. Stressed out? Well, sure — he was trying to prove himself at the university to get hired permanently, the boys were a handful, and money remained a struggle. But the biggest stress was this mysterious, debilitating illness. Regina had been reading up on his symptoms online and thought they pointed to a kidney problem. The doctor said she doubted it, the pain was too low in his back. But Regina insisted on an MRI.

A few days later, the doctor slid a CD of the scan into her computer, looked at the image, picked up the phone, and called the Hollidays. She said, I'd like to get you an appointment with an oncologist.

Time Stands Still

In room 109 of Washington Home and Community Hospices, Fred planned his funeral, determined not to leave Regina with a mess. He controlled his Dilaudid drip with the press of a thumb. Regina noticed that he rarely fingered the button when he had visitors. Whether he wanted to stay more alert or the company kept the pain at bay, she did not know.

For Regina, time seemed to stop. The more she thought about Fred's treatment before hospice, the angrier she became. She wanted to tell the world their story so experiences like theirs would not be repeated. During his second week in the hospice, she painted a mural called *Medical Facts* on a wall in a local deli. It showed a large skeleton beside a chart full of facts about his condition — a chart that looks like the nutrition labels on food. Her point was that patients and their caregivers should have full, easy access to information that can help them make the best decisions about care. Once she finished the piece, she began to make sketches for a large outdoor mural.

Relatives from around the country came to see Fred, and friends from every chapter in his life. His university buddies visited

172

regularly. They had seen him in the hospitals, listless as a ragdoll. Now, he seemed like the Fred they knew. He quoted poetry and whole scenes from the movie *Magnolia*. He told jokes. "He could be himself for the last month of his life," said his friend David Keplinger. Fred mentioned dying only once, telling David and Michael not to get upset or dwell on it but to enjoy the time they all had together. Both friends felt he said it more to put them at ease by verbalizing the unspoken reality than to get something off his chest. "Hospice seemed to be a relief in many ways," Michael said later. "Fred was finally getting the kind of treatment that seemed to make a difference in his day-to-day, moment-to-moment well-being."

Regina agreed. "He had a better quality of life in those last four weeks than at any other time because of the way he was treated. He was treated with dignity and respect and given the correct palliative care.

"The only problems arose when insurance people butted their heads in."

While Fred's turnaround brought joy to his family, it signaled to his health insurance company that he was strong enough to go home. After eleven days in the hospice, a discharge planner explained it to Regina.

Fred was not on Medicare, as Art Buchwald had been, but most private plans impose the same rules and limitations on service. They cover inpatient hospice care only until a patient is stable enough to be cared for at home.

"I can't take him home!" Regina protested. Their one-bedroom apartment was tight under the best of circumstances, and these were the worst. Fred's mother, Joan, had moved in to help with the kids. The place had no spare square foot for oxygen equipment, a hospital bed, and whatever else Fred would need. Nor could the family afford to hire help. Hospice would send a nurse every other day and an aide on alternate days, but that left Regina to handle everything the other twenty-three hours.

The hospice folks empathized — they knew the drill. "Families are always surprised when we say we have to send the patient home," said Beverly Paukstis, a registered nurse and director of hospice operations at Washington Home and Community Hospices. "They want to stay, and they're always shocked when they can't, even though it says it in the contract they signed." Paukstis sighed, a long "rules are rules" breath of resignation and irritation. She had worked in hospices since 1985, soon after Medicare started covering the services — creating the template for benefits that both the government and most private insurers use to this day. "We always say the Medicare hospice benefit was written by men who had housewives at home to take care of them."

Regina pleaded for time, called the manager of her apartment complex, and lucked out. A two-bedroom apartment had just opened up. She posted an appeal online for help and early one morning, friends and members of her church arrived at her apartment and packed it up. A week later, another crowd hauled boxes and furniture to the new place, down the hall, and set up a room for Fred. It had bookcases on three walls, with books and DVDs organized just the way he liked. The side of the bed faced a window, so he would be able to lie there and look outside.

Fred was transported to the new apartment the next day, Thursday, June 11. It felt like home. And that stressed everybody.

Isaac clung to Fred. Freddie shut himself in the other bedroom and came out only when Regina coaxed. Fred worried that Isaac would trip on a tube or wire, and Regina worried that the kids would accidentally hurt Fred. A nurse brought the hospice emergency kit, full of powerful drugs, and instructed Regina to store it in the refrigerator. "I'm not doing that. I have little kids, and this stuff is toxic," Regina said. She placed it on a high shelf in the linen closet.

Regina did laundry almost constantly — Fred's sheets, pillowcases, and pajamas. Her arms turned black and blue from lifting and turning him. On Sunday, Fred's third day home, a hospice nurse came, saw the turmoil in the household and the toll on Regina, and suggested transferring him back to the facility.

"Wait," Regina said. "How can I do that? I was told we had to leave."

That's how it works, the nurse said. You go home for three days and prove to insurance you can't handle it, and then you can come back.

Regina was furious. "You're telling me I moved my entire family and we got a year's lease on a new apartment because we needed to have Fred home and it really wasn't really the case?" And then she said no, Fred would stay home. She had promised him no more transports.

On Monday, his pain increased and he had trouble swallowing. That frightened him and panicked his mother, Joan. She wanted to call 911, which hospices discourage; even if patients have signed a "do not resuscitate" order, the emergency medical technicians may insist on trying to restart the heart or breathing, and things get complicated. Regina called the hospice nurse instead. She came quickly, adjusted Fred's medications, and spent a long time talking privately with Joan.

Tuesday around midnight, Fred's catheter slipped out. The nurse came again, and inserted one so efficiently that he complimented her. She then walked into the kitchen, picked up a broom, and began sweeping the floor. "You don't have to do that," Regina said.

"We're here to help you too," the nurse replied.

Fred wanted to talk with Regina. He rambled, meandering from Stephen King to Jon Stewart to the children. Around six o'clock in the morning, he looked at his wife and seemed to really see her. "Reggie, you look so tired," he said, lucidly. "You should go to sleep." She dozed for an hour and got up to give him his medicine. His eyes remained shut and he said nothing. She tried to rouse him and at last he opened his mouth and swallowed the crushed pills.

Then his breathing turned shallow. Joan said she was worried. Regina ran into the other bedroom and hustled the boys to Fred's side. Joan and Freddie held one hand. Regina and Isaac held the other. Fred died June 17, six days after leaving the hospice.

Eight days later, early in the morning, Regina squeezed paints onto her palette, climbed a twelve-foot ladder, and started painting a mural about Fred's health care experience. Her canvas was a twenty-foot high brick wall on the side of a BP gas station on busy Connecticut Avenue, overlooking the parking lot of a CVS Pharmacy. She had sold Fred's car to the guys at the gas station while he was sick. She'd noticed the wall then, and they said she could have it.

She had sketched the mural during long, quiet days in the hospice, rolling out long sheets of paper right there in the lobby. A few of the nurses served as models. She photographed them in workaday positions, standing, sitting, leaning over patients, or checking computer monitors, to capture the tilt of a head, the bend of an elbow, the drape of scrubs.

Regina painted all summer, as an outlet for her grief and her anger. Crowds gathered and cheered her on. Congress was debating President Obama's health reform plan at

178

the time, and a young, articulate widow making art across town about the health care system at its worst — fragmented, insensitive to the point of callousness, bureaucratic — proved irresistible to reporters. Her project was featured in the alphabet soup of media, including CNN, CBS, BBC, AOL, NPR, and the august *BMJ*, the *British Medical Journal.* It would mark the start of a new career for Regina as a patients' rights advocate, lecturer, and blogger.

Regina titled the mural *73 Cents,* because at the height of Fred's illness she asked to obtain a copy of his medical record and was told she would have to pay that sum, per page. The record ran to hundreds of pages.

On a cold night four months after Fred died, eighty people gathered to dedicate the mural. In its center, he lies stretched on a hospital bed, his eyes closed in slumber. In front of him is Regina with two faces in profile, like yin and yang. The face looking at Fred wears a mask like those cheap ones kids wear on Halloween, with the cutout eyes and flimsy elastic band. The mask has a radiant smile. Fred cannot see Regina's other face, gray and sagging in fatigue. It is looking away from Fred, toward a nurse, who ignores Regina and focuses instead on a blank computer screen. Nearby, a white-coated doctor is talking on a cell phone and, like the nurse, seems oblivious to the human need in the room. Another doctor, in scrubs, is tied up with red tape and standing in medical waste.

The Holliday boys are featured too. Isaac, with blond hair, wide blue eyes, and a half smile, sits cross-legged in the foreground. His is the only face looking straight at the viewer, in a gaze both innocent and challenging. Part of Freddie's face — a thatch of hair, an eye, part of a nose and mouth — appears in a thin strip of light color set against the dark brick wall. He seems to be peeking in, too scared to enter. Toward the top of the mural is a white clock with black numbers but no hands, a symbol of how time seemed to halt for the family while the rest of the world kept going.

Scattered through the mural are quotes from Hamlet, the Harry Potter books, Thomas Jefferson, and of course *Buffy*, Fred's favorite TV show and the inspiration for his doctoral dissertation. In its dark, quirky way, *Buffy* also inspired Regina to tell Fred's story through her art. "*Buffy* was not afraid to talk about dying," she wrote on her blog. "Dying was part of life. What really matters is how we live while we are here, how we treat others, and how important it is to stand up for what is right, even if it is hard." On the mural, a long white banner hangs from the ceiling of Fred's hospital room, and Buffy's words ring out: "Don't sing me songs. Give me something to sing about."

■ ■ ■ ■ ■

PART THREE:
THE SURVIVORS

■ ■ ■ ■ ■

CHAPTER EIGHT:
UP FROM THE ABYSS

"Are you still grieving?"

Picture a faintly lighted office with a somewhere-on-the-seaside painting the only spot of color, and think about gearing yourself up to spend an hour and a half with eight or ten strangers who, like you, recently lost the love of their life. The Birch Room lies just off the lobby at the Hospice of the Valley, a two-story brick building in San Jose. There are cookies, coffee, tea, and tissues, but office bones poke through earth-toned décor.

Bereavement services are hospice's best-kept secret. Even people who are familiar with the hospice concept are surprised by the wealth of support offered to people who are grieving, whether or not their loved ones used hospice. And while grief support has become a commercial industry, only in hospice is it an organic expression of the mission to embrace the whole family. Hospice founders recognized that loved ones may need attention long after the patient is gone, and that everyone benefits from care that helps them remain productive members of society. Free or low-cost, hospice-sponsored bereavement care varies in depth and quality, but it is not an add-on. It is part of the package.

Marilyn Anderson, fifty-five, did not think that part of the package was for her. The first Wednesday in November 2007, she walked into the Birch Room and knew right away she shouldn't have come. She had promised the hospice social worker she would give it a try, but as ten lost souls settled into the sofa and chairs nestled around a coffee table, Marilyn's first thought was: "I have nothing in common with these people."

Initially, they all felt that way. Nobody wanted to make new friends or hear other people's sad stories. But they were having trouble sleeping, eating, concentrating, and making simple decisions. Some were angry at being abandoned, depressed and remorseful about their loved one's suffering, anxious about not being able to handle life on their own. They never thought they'd be in a group like this, but they had to do something. The death of a husband or wife is well known to increase the risk of death for the surviving spouse.

In one way, Marilyn was right about being different from the rest. She was the only gay person in the room. Yet her second thought was: "These people look like I feel."

Marilyn had counted on dying first. Her partner, Irene Ringer, was eight years older, but Irene was the healthy one. Marilyn had long suffered from asthma and pulmonary sarcoidosis, painful inflammation of her lungs. She often had trouble breathing.

Irene, sixty-three, got headaches from time to time, but who doesn't? Stress, they both thought. All three of Irene's children were getting divorced. One morning, Irene put on her favorite outfit for the hospital office where they both worked, went to her computer, and did not know what to do. Marilyn reminded her how to log in. When Marilyn came back to check, Irene had not begun typing. She started to say something and no words came. They went to the emergency department, fearing a stroke.

A CT scan showed a small, irregular mass in her brain. Then, an MRI revealed more tumors and a biopsy confirmed: stage 4 glioblastoma, the most aggressive malignant brain tumor. She might live a few months, but only if she stayed in the hospital and underwent a multitude of invasive treatments.

After ten days of chemotherapy and radiation, with no progress and only the promise of more pain, Irene said to Marilyn and any doctor who would listen, "What is the point?" A couple for twenty-one years, they had talked about what they wanted at the end of their lives. Marilyn knew Irene hated any thought of being a sick person controlled by strangers. Now she kept saying, "What is the point? I want to go home."

But Irene's radiation oncologist said the hospital could not discharge her unless she could walk. They lived in a small below-market condominium jammed with musical instruments and sound equipment for Marilyn's playing in community orchestras. The bedroom was upstairs. Irene could hardly walk, let alone climb the narrow staircase.

Marilyn spoke daily with the next-door neighbors, whose family had used Hospice of the Valley. They set up a meeting in the hospital.

Irene got out of bed and dragged one foot in front of the other out the door. It would be the last time she ever walked.

Two hours after the discharge was OK'd, they were home. The neighbors had cleared out the living room so that hospice staff could bring in a hospital bed, a walker, and a commode. Medicines for pain, seizures, and blood pressure would be delivered. A hospice nurse came that day. Marilyn only had to buy bed sheets. It was a profound relief for both of them to have the stage set so they could focus on keeping Irene comfortable.

Hand-painted "Welcome Home, Grandma" posters and their little blond mutt, Epi, greeted Irene. She began to relax, in and out of consciousness for five days. Marilyn played her partner's favorite music. Irene had a stream of visitors, and her best friend flew in from Florida. She held their hands, smiled, and said, "Thank you. This is what I wanted. Bless your heart."

On the sixth day, a hospice nurse let Marilyn know death was near. Marilyn was singing from *The King and I,* "You may be as brave / as you make believe you are," when Irene died in bed.

Hospice of the Valley kept in touch with Marilyn, letting her know their services were not limited to preparing the patient and loved ones for death. Founded in 1979, Hospice of the Valley is the region's oldest nonprofit hospice. As required by Medicare, the hospice offers thirteen months of bereavement services free to families of their patients, on a sliding scale to the community, to help them through the first anniversary of death. There are workshops, memorial events, support groups for teenagers and people who've lost loved ones to suicide. A large playroom for children is stocked with a sand tray and toy figures, a dollhouse, and hand-painted facemasks on the walls.

At first, Marilyn declined — she never was comfortable sharing her emotions with anyone but Irene. But as weeks went by, Marilyn couldn't face work and had to take a leave. She felt she was suffocating. When she felt herself reverting to the recluse she had been before meeting Irene, she agreed to try the group.

On the Day the Morning Glories Bloomed

Introductions began with the man next to Marilyn, Phil Hamister, forty-nine, a buttoned-down Silicon Valley engineer. Stoic in the best of times, Phil couldn't eat or sleep after his wife's horrific death.

Six years earlier, he had found the love of his life in his second marriage. Then, alone at home on June 4, 2007, Gena, a vibrant fifty-year-old high-tech executive turned family therapist, collapsed. She dragged herself to the phone. An ambulance took her to the local hospital, but with the possibility of an aneurysm she was transferred to the trauma center at Stanford Hospital, half an hour away. Surgery stabilized the pressure on her brain, and doctors implanted a stent to divert fluid to her stomach.

Gena came out of it weak and changed, almost childlike — from the drugs or brain damage, they didn't know yet. It was a miracle she was still alive, doctors told Phil. After a week, she was sent home with loads of medications, and instructions that she not be left alone.

Two weeks later, Gena got up from a chair in the living room, crying in pain, and started for the bed. She fell and went into convulsions. Phil called 911, but even before the ambulance came, he knew it was another aneurysm and felt she was gone. Her face was blank. At the hospital, she was immediately hooked up to a ventilator. All night, as Phil held her hand and stroked her head, he spoke gently, "You are my angel, my princess. I love you."

The next morning, a battery of tests found no signs of life in Gena's brain. A doctor came in and told Phil that they had to make a decision. Phil talked with Gena's friends and family, waiting outside, but they all knew she'd never want to live this way. Phil doesn't remember the technician saying a word, just the tube whipping around on the bed like something alive, as the family watched in horror. Then all that was left was to listen to the beeping heart monitor and watch Gena's unchanging face. It took her twelve minutes to die.

Phil's daughter Laura drove him home. The morning glories he had planted and checked every day for any sign of flowers had chosen this day to bloom. Maybe it was a sign, Laura said, that life goes on.

But Phil felt only anger. He could not get past the final image of Gena — empty eyes wide open, her face contorted in pain. She was the social one, with lots of friends; he was the loner. Now he had nobody to talk to. Always physically active, a triathlete, he couldn't drag himself to run a mile. He spent hours at the cemetery. Just to make more time go by, he took the train to work instead of driving. Analytical by training and temperament, Phil cried every day. Finally, he went to see a therapist, who suggested the bereavement group. He had started the Wednesday after Labor Day, so by the time Marilyn arrived in November, he knew the ropes.

What Happens in Group, Stays in Group

The therapist, Bridget Flynn, made sure they always met in the same room, with the brown furniture in the same formation, the same tea and decaf coffee. At thirty-three, Bridget was a young mother and wife. Throughout her childhood, however, she had been around people in mourning. Her aunt and uncle ran a family funeral home. And when her grandmother died, Bridget went to live for several months with her bereft grandfather. She had learned that, in the chaos of grief, survivors crave consistency. Her job was to provide the space and let the group lead, following a Native American concept about every loss requiring a thousand tellings.

Besides cookies and tea, the people who gathered in Hospice of the Valley's Birch Room got a sheet of paper when they joined: Listening and Sharing Guidelines. Rules ranged from confidentiality ("Everything discussed in the group stays with the group") to sociability ("Encourage yourself to connect with group members between sessions") to manners ("Participate as fully as you can" but "Be careful about monopolizing time").

Marilyn could not imagine ever monopolizing time. Here she was, the Plain Jane among polished nails and coiffed hair. But when her turn came, she burst into tears and sobbed, "I'm sorry, my partner was a woman!" She had been a strictly Don't Ask/Don't Tell lesbian up to now. Between tears, Marilyn continued, "I don't even feel like I should I be here. I don't know what you're going to think of me. I can't take anymore, because it's all hurting."

Group members took turns saying the gay thing didn't matter at all. Marilyn drove home crying, but she returned the following week.

Phil's tendency, like Marilyn's, was to scan the room for all the ways other people were not like him. There were Shirley Gregory and Jerry Farnsworth, well into their sixties. They might have contemporaries who'd lost their spouses. Phil didn't. Was his loss more tragic? Also, most of the others had partners die after a long illness. His had happened in seconds. Finally, nobody else was an engineer, a species famously better at computation than emotion, Phil knew.

The differences receded as the stories continued. Phil liked that he could talk or just listen. And they were talking about the only subject he cared about. Soon enough, the Birch Room felt more comfortable than anyplace else in his life.

Bridget began each meeting with a two-minute meditation or reading about loss, and then: "Did anyone have anything happen this week that you want to share with the group?" She would tease out a theme — guilt, fear of the future, insensitive neighbors — and direct the discussion around that.

Bessie Williams, a widow at fifty-three, came into the group with some bad feelings about hospice. She had not gotten adequate instruction on pain medication in the awful final days of her husband, Tim. She needed to talk and, like Phil, felt utterly alone. Bessie had come to the United States when she was twenty-six, leaving her family in the Philippines. Her husband's family consisted of a sister in Washington state.

Bessie had tried three different spousal bereavement groups before finding the right fit. One was too small, with just four widows. One was too big, with little opportunity to talk. In the third, she just didn't feel a connection. Finally, in the Birch Room, the group clicked. As Bessie said later, "Some people are probably like, 'Good riddance! Thank God he's died, now I can really move on.' " In this group, everyone seemed to have loved their spouses very much.

In Bridget Flynn's spouse bereavement

groups, people usually bring in a photo of their partner by the second or third week. They soon start talking about "first times" doing something without them. By the fourth or fifth week, Bridget shifts the spotlight away from idealizing their spouses and gets to questions like: Am I ever allowed to feel good? And later: What am I missing? Sex, for example. When is it time?

Nobody went to the group looking for love, just a place to talk. And to keep talking, perhaps saying the same things over and over. Friends, family, and coworkers usually have limited capacities as sounding boards. They may avoid talking about grief at all, get impatient with it, or get very worried if it goes on too long. Everyone is afraid of saying the wrong thing, and we desperately want our loved ones to get better. In the group, nobody even suggested, as Bessie put it: "We've heard this already. Your turn is over. Next!"

Every year, nearly one million people in the United States lose their spouses. More lose a parent — a sad experience, but often anticipated and shared with siblings. Even when the death of a spouse or life partner is long expected, grief is intensely personal and different with each person. Just as

Americans think we're never going to die, we think our spouses won't either. And then, all of a sudden he has glioblastoma, surgery, chemotherapy, and radiation. He goes from a walker to a wheelchair to a hospital bed. At best, it ends in a death with dignity.

But hospice continues. The same questions may surface: What should I expect? What is normal? Survivors still may need the comfort and reassurance of calm, knowledgeable people who have been through this before. Group leaders like Bridget know, for example, that spouses often feel guilty, believing that they should have been better caretakers, that there were symptoms they should have caught, that their partners were perfect.

When someone in the Birch Room asked: "If you had that last day to do over would you change anything?" Bessie, who looks like Natalie Wood would have if she'd lived into her fifties, had a lot to say. "If I knew then what I know now, I would have called hospice a lot sooner." She didn't realize that Tim qualified for Medicare that would cover hospice. Swept up by the specialists' expertise and hopes for a cure, Tim endured horribly painful experimental chemotherapy. She would have said no to all that.

Everyone had stories of well-meaning friends, neighbors, and relatives saying something like, "Are you still grieving?" Or giving unwanted advice. "You're looking well" also was hard to take. In her memoir, *A Widow's Story,* Joyce Carol Oates recalls an overload of Sympathy Gift Baskets packed with gourmet food, and intrusive comments that were odd at best. An acquaintance: "Ohhh Joyce — you're wearing pink. How nice." A stranger: "My husband died ten years ago. It doesn't get any easier."

As Bessie would put it, "They don't know what they're talking about." She felt adrift in a harsh new world. She was a widow. Who was that, again? But listening to others' stories, Bessie felt, "Oh my goodness, life goes on." She would never forget Tim, but was heartened to hear Bridget say that people who had good marriages tended to welcome the idea of sharing their life again.

Besides the deep questions like "Who am I without my partner?" discussions also touched on practical matters. When a spouse dies, the paperwork of insurance and settling estates feels endless, and it's all yours, as is getting leaky faucets fixed or shopping for groceries.

Bessie liked learning what other people went through — in a venue that had completely different rules from anywhere else in life. They could say something mean about an aunt who was well intentioned but clueless. They could say nothing. Instead of worrying about when they might burst into tears, they could just do it. Having started where most relationships take years to grow into, they dispensed with a lot of pretense.

Phil began to schedule his life around the group meetings, the only place he felt safe. At work or while driving, he'd think, "Six days until group, five days until group . . ." Before Valentine's Day 2008, Phil had an idea about doing something for the women. He had a romantic side, but he checked first with Bridget to make sure that sending all the women flowers wouldn't cause more pain. One night, Bessie was floored to find two dozen long-stemmed roses sitting on her porch. She thought, "Who would send me flowers? I just lost my husband! And who were these men's names on the card? They must be guys Tim used to work with, but, on second thought, no, they wouldn't do that."

When she realized who they were, she called them all. She still has the card signed by Jerry, Phil, Billy, Chuck, and Ted.

"What Have I Got to Lose?"

Spousal loss groups at Hospice of the Valley run for six weeks and then take two weeks off. A few people dropped out or moved away, and new people joined.

Pamela Hammer joined in the spring, this group's third session. Her husband, Rusty, died January 28, 2008, after six months in hospice care. He'd had five years of aggressive treatment for leukemia, including a stem cell transplant. The Hammers had deep roots in the community but, as Pamela found, their friends had work to do and families to tend. And she wanted her children, recent college graduates, to get on with their own lives. She had let go of her real estate career to care for Rusty and wasn't ready to go back. What to do with the days?

Normally a social person, Pamela sat alone in the house where Rusty died. She knew she had to talk to someone, so when Hospice of the Valley called to offer bereavement counseling, she figured, "What have I got to lose?"

The woman she was assigned to for individual counseling was younger than Pamela's children. What could she possibly know about losing your partner of thirty-three years? Also, she specialized in art therapy and had Pamela cutting pictures and words out of magazines, feeling silly. But it triggered conversation and new perspectives. When, after a few months, the counselor suggested a group might be beneficial, Pamela asked, "But can't I stay with you?" Still, she agreed to give the group three tries.

That Wednesday night in April, Pamela sat next to Marilyn and began crying. Marilyn touched her hand to comfort her, and Pamela grabbed it and held on. Marilyn started feeling self-conscious. Being an out lesbian was so new; she worried what people just joining the group would think. She patted Pamela's hand and took her own back.

In later sessions, Pamela talked about her son's anger at his father for dying. Rusty worked so hard all his life, and his son wondered if his immune system was weak when he got cancer. The other group members with adult children understood perfectly, as well as their own anger at spouses who'd left them alone, which only made them feel worse. In the Birch Room, they found ways to untangle burdens that at first seemed impossible.

Meanwhile, Phil was becoming the group's unofficial social director. That spring, he suggested an outing to a local museum that most residents had never set foot in: the Rosicrucian Egyptian Museum and Planetarium in San Jose. It seemed an odd choice, a full city block of artifacts from ancient Egyptian tombs, including mummies, coffins, and texts detailing practices to ensure the afterlife. Then again, why not? Most of them had nothing else to do. Afterward the group went for lunch at a nearby coffee shop, where two of the older members, Jerry Farnsworth and Shirley Gregory, spoke directly to each other for the first time. Jerry sat next to Shirley and they had a strained conversation about the mummies. But unlike in other social situations, Jerry didn't feel like a fifth wheel.

Going back to work was harder for some. Federal law does not mandate that companies provide paid leave for bereavement. Many do, usually three days for a death in the immediate family — time to attend the funeral, basically. Some employers are more flexible about unpaid leave for people who are grieving, but the general attitude is that you shake yourself off and get back in the game.

For Marilyn, going back was particularly difficult because she and Irene had worked in the same hospital office. Everyone knew Irene as the fun one, Marilyn the shy one — except for co-workers who weren't sure which woman was which. After it was announced that Irene had died, one of the doctors asked, "Was she the nice one?" Marilyn had to think, "Actually, yes, she was."

Marilyn had studied violin in college, played harp, and performed in musical theater orchestras. Since Irene's illness, she had been unable even to look at the jumble of musical instruments in her living room — piano, guitar, Jew's harp, modern orchestra harp, and ukulele. Six months after starting the hospice group, though, she signed up for another show. When she mentioned this to the group, somebody asked, "Well, can we come?" And they did, giving Marilyn a whole row of familiar faces.

Cleaning out their spouses' things took a long, long time. Marilyn had to make a stab at it, because her sister was coming to visit with her husband and kids, and the place was a mess. Pamela, Shirley, Jerry, and another group member came over and spent five hours helping her clean out the garage, so she could make room in the house for guests.

Hospice bereavement group members are encouraged to get together socially. Dating, not so much. It can be a rebound relationship or what therapists call a "flight to health" by people so desperate to be normal again that they latch on before they really know what they want or need.

Bessie didn't worry about all that. She liked to bring people together, and took an interest in Jerry Farnsworth. A retired human resources manager, Jerry was the one person who came into group knowing that someday he wanted to date again. He was active in his Mormon church but hadn't met anyone there. When he asked Bessie: "Where do you meet someone?" she had already been thinking on his behalf.

"Maybe you should just look within the walls of the room where we are every Wednesday." He had noticed Shirley, and enjoyed talking with her at the Egyptian museum, but at group meetings when Bridget brought up the subject of getting married again, Shirley said she just couldn't see it. That made Jerry afraid to call her. Bessie got his permission to make the call for him. "What do you think about going out with Jerry?" she asked Shirley, who said, "Well, that would be nice."

Shirley, trim and attractive, and Jerry, quiet and athletic, both had been married forty-five years when their spouses died. They had married their high school sweethearts the same year, 1961. Shirley was living with her daughter's family. When Jerry came to call, he felt like he was back in high school. Shirley's son-in-law came to the door, and Jerry felt like saying, "Um, can Shirley come out and play?"

At first, group members got together just to get out of the house, as with going to work, except that they didn't have to make small talk or say thank you when someone said, "You're doing so well!" They got into the habit of going to at least one social event each month. It could be a carefully vetted movie, dinner, bowling, or a baseball game. They celebrated birthdays — their own and sometimes their partner's.

One day they were playing bocce ball and Marilyn noticed something astonishing: "You know what? We're laughing. We're laughing!"

CHAPTER NINE: TURNING POINTS

"You're still hurting, but you want that love in your life."

It could start with a laugh. Research confirms the importance of laughter in reducing the stress of bereavement. But, after losing the one person who was always there, how do you know that you really are climbing out of the abyss? Turning points don't announce themselves. People who keep journals have something to hold in their hands and remind themselves that a few months ago they couldn't get out of bed, let alone laugh, but absent a written record it's hard to see how things have improved.

In the Birch Room at Hospice of the Valley, Phil Hamister, Marilyn Anderson, and the other spouses in the bereavement group heard and re-heard one another's stories of loss into their second year. But the tone changed. Maybe their spouses had some faults worth mentioning. Everyone spoke less about health problems, now that their eating, exercise, and sleep had improved. They were better able to focus at work. They made plans and went out, often with one another. Eventually there would be romance but for now, it was mainly group-initiated outings. They chose places that wouldn't be laden with memories.

Phil organized a ferry ride across San Francisco Bay, an excursion none of them had done with their spouses.

It was a blue-sky day on the bay, with just a little breeze. But while the rest were together on the boat, Marilyn tried to mingle in a restaurant on the pier, feeling left out. She had committed to a birthday party with her next-door neighbors, whom she loved and would always appreciate for connecting Irene with hospice. This Sunday, the restaurant was buzzing with two dozen relatives and friends clinking glasses and talking over each other. Before dinner was served, Marilyn gazed out a panoramic window at the bay, where the people she treasured most at this moment likely were having a great time without her. A half-hour into the birthday festivities, she saw a ferry approaching and called Bessie. No answer — they probably couldn't hear their phones through the ferry's horns. Then Bessie texted back: The ferry was coming in right then. She should come meet them.

Even in her happiest times with Irene, nobody thought of Marilyn as spontaneous. That was Irene's department. On back to childhood, Marilyn never would have done what Bessie was suggesting: Leave the people she had come with and go chase a ferry. But now, who cared? Marilyn excused herself and said, "I'm going to meet some friends. I'll be right back."

It had been only a few days since she'd seen the group, but everyone waved madly, as if they were the parents and Marilyn was coming home from college. There were hugs all around, and quick reports of the day. After twenty minutes, Marilyn walked back to the restaurant and through the busy dining room, with a big smile on her face. One of the family asked, "What happened to you?" She felt as if she had just won a big award.

The Possibility of a Future

Back in the Birch Room, group members spoke about the possibility of a future. As in: What are you looking for? What is your new life going to look like? Do you ever envision marrying again? For a long time they couldn't talk about their grief anywhere but here. Now the Birch Room was where they could talk honestly about the possibility of moving on.

Shirley Gregory had spent the first year talking about how she couldn't imagine ever remarrying, scaring Jerry Farnsworth away when she said, "I never thought I'd be alone. I thought we'd grow old together." Exactly like Jerry, she had married her high school sweetheart, and they'd been together forty-five years. Phil and Gena had been married only six years, and he felt the same way, that they would grow old together.

Shirley had a dream in which Jim, her dead husband, came back and talked to her, and she told him how badly she missed him. It was so vivid, she felt Jim's presence. Now, Shirley Gregory is no Shirley MacLaine. A real estate agent in her sixties, Shirley Gregory never dabbled in New Age spirituality and wasn't about to mention her strange dream to the neighbors. But she could tell the group about the conversation with her husband, and that she felt released in some way to enjoy life again. Nobody doubted her.

They no longer expected to see their wife in the mirror while brushing their teeth, or the phone to ring and hear their husband's voice. They were learning, as author Anne Roiphe wrote upon losing her husband: "I can read. I can think. I can work. I can see friends. I can watch my grandchildren grow. I can walk in the park and I can listen to music and I can argue politics and I can pass, if fate allows it, from old to older in the usual manner. I will be sad often but not always. I will be lonely most always but not unbearably so."

By the second year, everyone considered it "My Group." They had shed their politeness with each other, sharing unbecoming angers and fears. They were like family in that way, and in another way: They had been forced to work together on projects not of their own choosing. Like siblings grumbling about having to do the dishes, they faced a number of projects in the hospice's art room with eyes rolling. One day, they painted double-sided cardboard facemasks: how they thought their faces looked to the world versus how they felt inside. Then they talked about the gaps between their perceptions of themselves and one another.

Some started dating. A therapist might warn them about the dangers of rushing into another relationship, but hearing "Go slow" or "I did it, and it didn't work" from another group member could be easier to accept. Well-meaning friends and family might say, "Tim would want you to be happy again" or "You shouldn't feel guilty." But for bereaved spouses, to date or not to date would become less about guilt or what the dead would want, and more about rejoining the world.

"You're still hurting, but you want that love in your life," Pamela said. She met Bob Conroy, sixty-two, a retired county sheriff, the day they both joined the group. They started going out to dinner together, then dating, and then dealing with the shrines to their spouses. Pamela said to Bob, "I know you love Melanie, but there are about a thousand photos around the house. Can we take one or two down?" He agreed to do that, if she removed the giant blowup picture of Rusty in her office.

Bessie had a widower friend who'd dated a divorcée. It didn't work out, Bessie felt, because their losses were so different. When she and Phil started going out, there was a basic level of understanding and comfort. And, of course, they were attracted to each other.

For their first date, the inveterate match-maker and the serious engineer took a walk across the Golden Gate Bridge and had dinner at the Cliff House, a century-old San

Francisco landmark. These are must-dos for tourists, but many longtime residents, like Bessie and Phil, never get around to them. Bessie was coming to realize how much she had taken for granted before, that there would always be time to do new things.

Jerry and Shirley, neither of whom had ever dated anyone but the spouses they met in high school, would be the first to get married.

The Bereavement Backlash

Bereavement groups are not for everyone. Sometimes people have issues, like alcoholism, that would flood the group. Others do better in individual counseling, going to workshops or finding meaning in spiritual practices offered by hospice. Medicare requires hospices to offer grief services, but they are not specifically reimbursed. They vary in approach and quality.

At their best, bereavement services express three of hospice's basic values:

The patient and family constitute the unit of care.

Listening is an essential act of care.

Care continues for the family after the patient dies.

"Both facing loss and turning away are appropriate responses so long as they do not last too long," writes British psychiatrist Colin Murray Parkes, founding father of hospice bereavement care. Parkes met Cicely Saunders in 1966, and she invited him to start a bereavement service at St. Christopher's Hospice. Parkes found the key to be "the provision of a secure base in which people can feel safe enough" to face the pain of loss and move into the "restoration mode."

In recent years, hospices have added online grief healing discussion groups moderated by professional counselors. At Hospice of the Valley, groups have been so successful that they have been subdivided by age as well as type of loss. There's a group for people who've lost loved ones to suicide, for people who prefer art therapy to talking, and for people whose loss of a grandparent, for example, was natural, expected, yet painful nonetheless.

Beyond hospice, grief support is on offer from churches, psychiatrists and self-described experts. At www.grieving.com you can find grief groups devoted to coping with the holidays, violent death, and nuclear disaster in Japan. The San Francisco Society for the Prevention of Cruelty to Animals has sponsored weekly pet loss support groups since 1982, and now a website, www.petloss.com, tracks the support groups in every state.

All this attention to survivors has sparked a nasty backlash. In her 2011 book, *The Truth About Grief,* journalist Ruth Davis Konigsberg attacks "our modern grief culture," which promotes the belief that grief must be long and hard, and the only way out is to work through it — preferably by paying someone to help you. In 2008, the hospice industry paid 5,000 full-time employees in bereavement services, a number Konigsberg finds shockingly excessive. But 5,000 employees averages to one per hospice. At least 1 million Americans lose their spouses every year, so that would be one care worker for every 200 survivors, not to mention people who've lost children, parents, close friends, and other loved ones. A total of 2.5 million deaths occur in America every year, leaving about four times that many mourners. Recently bereaved people are at far higher risk of developing physical disease, of having accidents, of developing behavioral difficulties that hurt themselves and others.

Some see the pharmaceutical industry licking its chops over a change in the *Diagnostic and Statistical Manual of Mental Disorders,* which previously advised clinicians not to diagnose a major depressive disorder in the first two months following the death of a loved one. In the recent fifth edition, that "bereavement exclusion" is gone, prompting critics to charge that DSM-5 effectively says: "Take a pill to get over the death of your loved one." In fact, this may be more of a danger with physicians not extensively trained in death and dying, especially with elderly people already on multiple prescriptions. But a temporary course of an antidepressant may be just what's needed to keep the person from sinking lower. Many survivors, particularly widowers, don't bounce back. Parkes found repeated studies showing an increased mortality rate for widowers during the first year of bereavement. He writes, "Men are more likely than women to die of a 'broken heart.'"

Good hospice grief counselors know when mourners need a push, not just empathy. If a woman lost her husband unexpectedly in October, and in February she still can't believe it happened and is still talking as if he might come back, the Hospice of the Valley counselor may make a point of inserting "When your husband died . . ." into the conversation.

More than six months after their loss,

about 20 percent of mourners have trouble functioning, and may remain isolated and have suicidal thoughts. This is called complicated grief. For the vast majority, studies have found that companionship helps a lot. Which is why professionally led groups may be exactly right. Countering the common fear that all that grief will be overwhelming, well-run groups are not free-for-alls.

"No, it wouldn't be great if everybody shared every feeling. People don't share for good reasons," said Dale G. Larson, director of graduate studies in health psychology at Santa Clara University. Larson has written and spoken extensively about end-of-life care and led bereavement groups. "You ask: Are you having trouble with grief and loss? Do you want help? Here's what we can do."

Bereavement groups work because participants are motivated to be there, not recruited, and because people usually join a few months after the death has occurred. Pain is fresh but habits are malleable. And, they have not spent years ruminating about their loss.

Hospice bereavement care's connection with Swiss-born American psychiatrist Elisabeth Kübler-Ross also has drawn fire. The original grief guru, Kübler-Ross pioneered the concept of death as a natural stage of life in her 1969 game changer, *On Death and Dying.* Based on her care for and interviews with terminally ill patients, she introduced the instantly famous five stages: denial, anger, bargaining, depression, and acceptance. But the stages were widely misinterpreted as marching orders, and endlessly repurposed for all kinds of transitions in life. When the U.S. economy tanked in 2008, commodities guru Kevin Kerr cited Kübler-Ross: "Only time will tell if the United States can actually move into the acceptance stage." Kübler-Ross herself reapplied the five stages in her last book, *On Grief And Grieving,* which critics saw as overreaching. But even there she declared at the start that the stages "were never meant to help tuck messy emotions into neat packages. They are responses that many people have, but there is not a typical response to loss, as there is no typical loss. Our grief is as individual as our lives."

Life Goes On

By the end of their second year, the summer of 2009, most of the group had said goodbye to the Birch Room. Marilyn and Phil, whose partners had died so quickly, tried a third year, but then they too stopped coming. They didn't need it anymore.

"Hospice took me from the depths of hell, this barren wasteland, a world of grays and ashes, to kind of an understanding of what I was going through. It put me on a path to recover," Phil recalled in a coffee shop a year after leaving the group. "Marilyn and I, it took us the longest to right our ship. Now we are steering toward sunrise rather than oblivion."

Phil still suffered from insomnia. But he started training to do another triathlon. He and Bessie were a solid couple, having dated more than a year since their walk across the Golden Gate Bridge. And he had a calendar of events to attend. Besides dinner, game nights, movies, and baseball games, the group had established a tradition for the Fourth of July, Christmas, and New Year's Eve. And then there was a wedding. The invitations read:

Our fondest wish is to be
Surrounded by the love of family
And friends at our wedding on
Valentine's Day

Please join Shirley and Jerry on
February 14th, 2010
5:30 p.m.

It was a small wedding at Shirley's daughter's house, with lots of grandchildren running around, a handful of old friends, and nine members of the hospice group.

Soon, Pamela and Bob went hiking, biking, and horse-riding in Utah with Jerry and Shirley. Pamela also became Shirley's partner in a real estate firm.

Meanwhile, Marilyn was having a hard time, especially when the holidays came around. She'd only learned to tolerate the Christmas season through years with fun-loving Irene. But then something someone had said about the holidays occurred to her, something helpful, and it bothered her that she couldn't quite place it. She talked to Phil, who remembered the thought had come from Bridget. For Marilyn, it was like having a brother who said, "Yeah, remember when Mom and Dad said . . ." The group had planted seeds. Some, like Phil's morning glories, took their time germinating.

Phil Hamister and Bessie Williams got engaged on September 27, 2011. They had planned to be in Chicago for Bessie's birthday, and he made dinner reservations at the top of the Hancock Building, famous for its panoramic views from ninety-four floors up. Phil bought a diamond ring and secretly ordered Champagne. But it wasn't going the way he planned. Bessie was glued to the window, exclaiming, "Look at those pools! Look at the breakwater!" Phil started to sweat. Finally, he got down on bended knee. This, she noticed, and said, "Yes, of course!" After dinner, he had arranged for a horse and carriage ride around Chicago, back to their hotel.

A few months later, Bessie had a herniated disc requiring emergency surgery. Then Phil's sister died, and he got laid off. Phil is the guardian of his disabled nephew. In the summer of 2012, Shirley shared terrible news. Jerry's oldest grandson had died at nineteen.

The group knew to offer help with errands and food, and to avoid hollow words or to trample on Jerry's private nature. Shirley asked for help with a memorial service in a friend's back yard. It was hot that day, but as they gathered around a big tree, a breeze came up and Marilyn played a hymn of resurrection from Handel's *Messiah,* "I Know that My Redeemer Liveth."

Pamela Hammer eventually moved into Bob Conroy's house and changed everything, from hardwood floors to new paint inside and out. They would be married in October 2013 at an inn overlooking Monterey Bay. Pamela's children were to light a candle for Rusty, and Bob's for Melanie. All their hospice buddies would be there.

The lost souls who had gathered warily in the Birch Room to try to reclaim their lives often wondered why so many couples came out of their group. Facilitator Bridget Flynn has a theory: "They were fearless, and so supportive of each other. They had such different personalities and backgrounds. If you'd put them together in any other situation, who knows if a relationship would have developed. Probably not."

What they had in common was a powerful love for their spouses, and a willingness to work hard to get that love back in their lives. As Bridget says, "I always told them they were very special. They'd say, 'Aw, you say that to all your groups.'"

••••

Part Four:
The Providers

••••

CHAPTER TEN:
THE GIFT OF GRACE

• "How can I help you?"

The patient in a New York City bone transplant unit said no, he did not want to see the chaplain. He was not religious. Across the country, in hospice care at home in San Diego, a man dying of lung cancer was wary about participating in some new tell-your-story program called Dignity Therapy — and his longtime partner really did not love the idea.

Both patients pushed aside doubts, took a leap of faith, and discovered a capacity to live, grow, and find joy until the moment they died.

They were offered these options because, unique in health care, attention to nonphysical needs is woven into the daily practice of hospice. It has been from the beginning. Hospice pioneers recognized that pain is not just a medical problem and that emotional, psychological, and spiritual distress can cause physical anguish. Easing that distress is integral to the healing that is possible when a cure is not.

The patient's first question may be, "Why has God abandoned me?" or just, "Why me?" In hospice, and increasingly in palliative and pastoral services in hospitals, spiritual care can ease the sense of abandonment behind that question. It tries to help patients feel connected — perhaps to God, a sense of transcendence, or maybe to other people or to their own younger, vibrant selves. The spiritual support of hospice may draw on the patient's religious background or on music, poetry, aromatherapy, yoga, the touch of a visiting pet, or a life review. The point is to regain a link to the world outside the dying body.

In the *Journal of Palliative Medicine,* researchers distilled the essence: "Healing is distinguished from cure in this context. It refers to the ability of a person to find solace, comfort, connection, meaning, and purpose in the midst of suffering, disarray, and pain."

When the patient in the New York transplant unit declined her help, Mychal Springer, a soft-spoken woman with dark curly hair, did not press. "OK," she said.

"I'm Rabbi Springer. I'm the chaplain. If you change your mind, let me know."

As she turned to walk away, he stopped her. "Wait a minute. Did you say rabbi? Well, OK, you can come back sometime."

Springer went back a lot. The man told her he had been raised Catholic. He was no longer religious but considered himself spiritual, and in the hospital he'd had a revelation about his life. He had treated people unkindly and he needed to change course. He seemed relieved to admit that, but the rabbi sensed that something else bothered him. One day, while she was there, a Eucharistic minister came by and offered to give the man communion.

"I can't take communion," he said, and the minister left.

Springer had heard the words "I can't" — not "I don't want to." She asked him why he could not take communion, and he said he had been divorced and remarried. She could feel the hurt that his separation from ritual and tradition caused him. Springer told him she knew a hip, open-minded nun he might like, and he consented to see her. Then the nun said she knew a priest whom the patient would love, and the priest visited. The priest granted the man absolution and gave him communion. The patient's wife took communion too, and they started planning a church wedding. Although he died before they could arrange it, their reconciliation with their religious community brought them both a sense of fulfillment and peace.

As director of the Center for Pastoral Education at the Jewish Theological Seminary in New York, Springer trains seminary students of diverse faiths to provide pastoral care to people with serious or terminal illnesses. "Part of being a chaplain is that you enter into somebody else's space," she said. "Especially when you're in a hospice chaplaincy and you go into people's homes and you say: How does your life make sense to you? How can I help you draw on your own tradition and on your own sense of what is spiritual? How can I help you take the next steps, whatever they are, to find religious coherence and a sense of meaning in *your* life?"

By enrolling in hospice, patients and families take the first step, of accepting that life will end. Once in hospice care, time and energy previously spent pursuing curative treatments has opened up. What to do with that time? Hospice offers choices, not a set of beliefs. The standard opening question from the spiritual care team is, as Springer asked: "How can I help you?"

Cicely Saunders posed this question from the beginning of the hospice movement, focusing on the patient as a whole person, with hopes and dreams beyond the body's disease. Other hospice tenets — notably, the family as the unit of care, the teamwork of the hospice staff, and the integration of volunteers — dovetail in fostering spiritual and emotional support. Saunders maintained that, even with terminal cancer patients, "Pain was not just a physical sensation; it might be a consequence of loneliness, spiritual distress, inappropriate diet, or tumor growth. Careful listening was the most important skill in determining the best way to reduce patient discomfort."

Early Christian literature laid the foundation. The *Ars Moriendi* ("art of dying") manuals dating from medieval times provided guidance for the dying about what to expect, the importance of companionship, paving the way for a "good death," such as: "When any of likelihood shall die, then it is most necessary to have a special friend, the which will heartily help and pray for him and therewith counsel the sick for the weal of his soul."

The Volunteer as "Special Friend"

Most of the people who visit dying patients have an agenda: the nurse with medications, the aide to bathe, the social worker negotiating a family conflict, the loved one who desperately wants the dying patient to eat something. The volunteer has no agenda but to listen, to be that "special friend."

More than 430,000 people volunteer at hospices across the country. For Medicare and Medicaid certification, federal law requires that at least 5 percent of patient care hours be provided by volunteers, to de-institutionalize hospice and keep it more humane. While the professional staff has tasks to accomplish, volunteers have time. They might take a dementia patient outside and give him the chance simply to look at a tree and feel a breeze.

The Zen Hospice Project in San Francisco runs one of the oldest and most prolific programs for volunteers, with more than 100 every year serving at a large public hospital and a small residential facility. Volunteers range in age from twenty to seventy-five. They complete forty-five hours of training in spiritual care for the dying, work five hours a week, and attend monthly meetings and two retreats a year. Volunteers practice "mindfulness" of the certainty of death with patients and within themselves, benefiting both. "You get to see: Ah, this is what the dying process can be about," said Roy Remer, who started as a volunteer and now manages the hospice facility. "I remember shifts when I'd be feeling under the weather, wasn't sure how long I'd stay, then I would leave my shift feeling so buoyant, even healed in some way, from what I received back from residents. Whether they've accepted, surrendered, or are very resistant, they're teachers for us because they're simply going before us. They're sorting it out."

Guest House room and board is not covered by Medicare. Patients may want to watch TV all day, or eat candy. A whiteboard in the kitchen keeps track: "Ruth is eating hot dogs, French toast, caramels. David is making a transition from solids to liquids."

Talking to a visitor at the hospice's Guest House one day, Remer excused himself to answer the door. "You're here to see Felicia, who's arriving," Remer softly told the man he recognized as Felicia's husband. With no sirens or car doors slamming, the newest resident at the immaculate five-bedroom Victorian had just been driven there and was now sitting on the back patio, in the sun. From that moment until her death in a high-ceilinged bedroom with dark wood furniture and a bed for her husband, everyone at the Zen Hospice would be devoted to the question: "How can I help you?"

The Need to Be Seen and Heard

For health care professionals, spirituality started gaining traction in the early 1990s, and by 2009 more than 85 percent of medical and osteopathic schools taught subjects related to spirituality. Degrees in nursing and social work also incorporate spirituality. Many religious denominations and theology schools require students to complete courses of clinical pastoral education, which involves work in hospitals with dying patients. "Their job may be to introduce the *d-word*," said a veteran hospital chaplain and educator.

All of this harks back to Medicare's original mandate that hospices provide spiritual care. The steps are very specific, starting with an assessment of the patient's and family's spiritual needs by someone on the hospice team. Questions may be: Do you consider yourself a religious or spiritual person? Do you identify with any faith or belief? What do you believe in that gives meaning to your life? Is there a person or group of people you really love or who are really important to you?

The hospice is then required to follow up, by contacting local clergy, pastoral counselors, or others who can support the patient's and family's spiritual needs.

In recent years Medicare reaffirmed this, including the requirement that even patients on hospice for only days, and those in the debilitating end-stage of disease, be asked right away about any spiritual issues, such as anger at God, and: "How would you like me, and your treatment team, to address these issues?"

Language gets tricky. God, for starters. At the 2011 Hospice Foundation of America conference, "Spirituality and End-of-Life Care," one panelist suggested a nonsectarian way to think: "God is in the quality of our devotion to God's creatures." Amid tables piled with brochures for mortuaries and funeral caterers, much discussion centered on the word *chaplain.* People generally connect chaplains with the military and tend to think of them as bearers of bad news. Some hospice chaplains prefer *spiritual care adviser.* One caregiver suggested *minister* might be less loaded, but others found that too religious, and definitely too Christian.

Had the three godmothers of hospice been in attendance, they too would have had trouble settling on the proper language. Cicely Saunders and Rose Hawthorne Lathrop were ardent Christians, but Florence Wald adopted a more humanist vision of spiritual care as embracing "a reverence for life."

Hospice chaplains may be ministers, priests, rabbis, imams, monks, and lay people. But they are identified leaders who have at least 1,600 hours of interfaith clinical pastoral education — as are hospital chaplains. All are trained to deal with people in crisis, to maintain therapeutic boundaries, and to work with patients of all faiths, beliefs, and doubts. One difference is that Medicare requires spiritual care providers to be an integral part of the hospice team, while hospital chaplains are not part of the main business of medical and surgical treatment.

For hospital chaplains, end-of-life discussions often occur in the ICU. In the twenty-five years that the Reverend C. George Fitzgerald has been doing spiritual care at Stanford Hospital, he has found that "people like to ignore death if they can, especially in a hospital." He added, "We're here to send them home, not to their eternal home." Fitzgerald directs the hospital's spiritual care services, and his staff may counsel a patient at the very end, help handle funeral arrangements, or be the only professional the patient can tell to go away.

Why talk to a stranger, anyway? Fitzgerald likened it to being on a cross-country flight with hours to talk about your spouse's infidelity to someone you'll never see again. Some clergy are better at giving sermons than talking one-on-one, just as some doctors are better at technology, and patients may worry about burdening their own clergyperson, just as they hesitate to burden family.

"Death and dying is such a taboo area, frightening area. People end up feeling inhibited, and the end result is that the person who's dying is left alone," said Linda Emanuel, director of the Buehler Center on Aging, Health and Society at Northwestern University. "The startling thing, it turns out, we're all human beings with a heart and an experience, and we all want to be heard, and we all have feelings about life and the people we're closely related to in this life." That's why Emanuel likes narrative therapies, particularly Dignity Therapy. "People often have a compelling need to 'write the last chapter' of their life work," she said.

The Art of Listening

Narrative therapies have evolved to meet that need. In the early 1960s, before hospice came to this country, Robert Butler, a pioneer of gerontology and a research psychiatrist, described a formal process for looking back on one's life. He saw the reminiscences of older people as a natural and productive process. It intensified as they neared death, when people often seized the opportunity to resolve issues before "the closing of the gates." He called it life review and devised a battery of interview questions to help patients in nursing homes to organize their thoughts — from when and where they were born to what they consider the hardest thing about growing older.

More recently, the research-based protocol called Dignity Therapy incorporated elements of psychotherapy, narrative, diary writing, end-of-life confessionals, and checklists. It made sense to Canadian psychiatrist Harvey Chochinov that Grandma and Grandpa liked to reminisce. Being elderly was a life-cycle role, like the child's role and the parent's role, and with medical advances this role's time span was increasing. But often the family got tired of hearing the same stories, and the elder just got more anxious. Chochinov devised a protocol, standardized to be easily replicated, to help people record meaningful aspects of their lives in a book that they can pass down to their survivors. Where life review focuses on facts, Dignity Therapy is more reflective, bridging the psychological, spiritual, emotional, and social issues that added up to Cicely Saunders's concept of "total pain."

Sometimes people want their families to know about their accomplishments — how they built up a business from scratch or raised four children on their own. Others have trouble getting started, sure that they have done nothing worth telling anyone about. The twelve basic questions of Dignity Therapy are designed to get them talking about what is meaningful, to help them die in peace and leave a tangible legacy.

Dignity Therapy can give dying patients the precious opportunity of a do-over. Lori Montross, a psychologist and Dignity Therapy researcher, recalled, "One man, after I read his document to him, said, 'Am I that cranky? Wow, I don't want to be like that.' And he made a decision: 'I'm *not* going to be like that.' "

The run-through with an interviewer sometimes prepares patients to have these conversations with a loved one, even before they get a copy of the book.

Patients select a title and a cover photo, which also can be a revelation. Montross had a patient she knew only as a frail old man in a wheelchair, but his cover photo was astonishing — a handsome Humphrey Bogart lookalike lighting a cigarette. The man had been a model, and this picture had been in *Life* magazine. "That's in part the value of Dignity Therapy," Montross said. "I was giving him the opportunity to be seen the way he wanted to be seen."

Dignity Therapy did not seem like a great idea to Lisa Amparan. She might find out something she did not want to know about the man she loved. But she also knew he needed to do something meaningful with the time he had left, for both of them.

They had been together for twenty-eight years. When Peyton "Pete" Dralle, seventy-two, was diagnosed with throat cancer, Amparan, forty-six, quit her job in medical marketing to care for him. Pete went thirty-five rounds with radiation and then a few months of tube feeding before settling into almost a year of decent recovery. He took the radiation oncologist's advice: "Got something to do? Just go do it."

Pete and Lisa drove north to see the

California Redwoods one more time together. Pete was organized with his business affairs, but now he made lists of passwords and other details that Lisa would need to know. An outgoing guy, Pete became friends with his speech therapist. Around Memorial Day 2010, the therapist jolted them by saying, "You really ought to be in hospice."

Pete was skeptical and sent the intake person from the hospice packing. Lisa called her back, and this time Pete found he liked what she was saying, including her easy banter about the sport he loved: golf. And then he liked everybody hospice sent, from the male nurse who, like Pete, came from North Carolina, to the spiritual counselor, a former nun who'd had "impure thoughts," as did Pete.

But when the nurse mentioned that hospice offered Dignity Therapy, as part of a research project, and that Pete might be a good candidate, it was Lisa's turn to reject the idea. Pete was a copious note-taker, kept journals, and liked to tell stories. He also liked the idea that his participation could help someone else. But Lisa freaked out. "Gosh, I really know this person inside out and upside down, I think, but — would there be some other woman?"

They knew each other's history. Both had

been married before, and when Pete got sick they committed to staying together without getting married. Their relationship was a little tangled. First, Lisa and Pete had been together, then he had another girlfriend, then he came back to Lisa. He still talked to that woman from time to time. He had lost touch with his four children but had some contact with grandchildren. He tried with his daughter, but nothing came of it. However, he was very close to his godson. He wanted to stay alive to see Grant go off to college.

But now Pete was so thin that he could not stand to look at himself in the mirror, and he did not know what to tell people who called or wanted to visit except, "Yeah, I'm still waiting to die. Gotta go!"

As Lisa said, "Dying left him with too much free time."

Making the Dignity Therapy recordings filled some of the empty hours, but the real payoff was that answering the questions helped Pete to focus. What did he want to do with the rest of his life? He and Lisa devised what they called a "cup list," a lot smaller than a bucket list, considering his waning health. One item was to have a final conversation with his former girlfriend. Another was to build birdhouses for the golf course Pete loved.

Lisa had never been a planner. More the freewheeling type, she imagined if she ever needed a lot of money she could win the Lottery. Now she thought: What if I get sick or lose my job? She started paying attention to the paperwork that Pete had always done so diligently. Years earlier, he had made a sales call that changed his life, at the apartment of an elderly woman. She had signed up for a six-dollar membership in the Auto Club of Southern California but could not get her hand to write the check. She finally said to Pete and his supervisor, "I want to tell you young people something. There's nothing you can do about getting old. But don't be old and poor."

Although Pete had never been a spendthrift, after that encounter he studied compound interest, redoubled his saving, bought the house where Lisa still lives, and paid off the loan. It all came back to him in responding to the Dignity Therapy question: What lesson have you learned in life that you would want to pass along?

"I can't imagine having $25,000 to $30,000 worth of credit card bills and having five or six credit cards. Like this house — it is paid for, and I have no reason to move. . . . I wanted to make sure I never outlived my money or my means."

Pete had other practical advice, like don't be a person who, "when all else fails, reads the instructions." (That spoke to Lisa.) But his answers also went deeper. When asked to talk about the times he felt most alive, Pete mentioned hiking to 11,500 feet in the Sierra Nevada, and then surprised everyone by saying, "I've also felt very alive in these last few months."

Why?

"Because each day has become so precious. I have good days, and I have some really bad days. So on the good days I feel really alive! Like one day I went up to play golf, and it was an especially good day. I remember when I was walking on the golf green, and I could feel the grass up through my feet. It was a brand new sensation."

What are your hopes and dreams for your loved ones?

He hoped they got what they wanted, not what he wanted. He hoped they stayed healthy. "I also hope that, for whoever reads this, they have a chance to fall in love. It is a feeling like no other."

Psychologist Lori Montross transcribed the interviews, brought them back to Pete for editing, and wrote a concluding note, "Here is a man offering a final gift of grace."

A month later, Pete and Lisa had a fifteen-page spiral-bound notebook to read.

Which, at first, neither wanted. He already knew everything in it, and she was afraid of what she might find about the other women. One day, they took the notebook to bed and read it together. Lisa felt relieved to find nothing she didn't know. She made a hard-cover copy, with clear protectors for pictures to highlight the stories.

Later they read it with their godson, Grant, and his teenage brothers, who were interested to learn that Pete had run away from home at seventeen and joined the Navy. Also, there was a reference to Pete's *Summer of '42* love affair. Pete and Lisa had to explain a bit about *Summer of '42* being an old movie about a teenager's romance with, um, a married woman.

Pete died peacefully on the living-room couch, on January 6, 2011.

A week later, his former girlfriend called Lisa and said she was leaving the area for a new job. She wanted to come by the house, where she had lived as well. As they sat in the living room, Lisa listened to the woman's life story. Had Pete talked about her? Not much, Lisa said. As Lisa understood it, "She just needed to do this before she moved on. We hugged and she went on her way." At last, Lisa was able to let go of her insecurities.

The Power of Prayer

Many people still want spirituality to be about God. While active participation in organized religion has ebbed in America, the country retains a deep vein of spirituality. Studies show that most patients want their health care providers to ask about spiritual concerns, and not only when they are about to die. Americans of every major religion as well as those unaffiliated with any religion also have a strong belief in miracles, and it influences how they think about life-threatening illness or injury. In one study, 61 percent of people surveyed said a miracle could save a person in a persistent vegetative state, while only 20 percent of trauma professionals agreed. Most people also said that divine intervention could save a person even if a doctor insisted that further treatment was futile.

Research shows too that most patients with a serious illness feel that the medical system does not adequately support their spiritual needs. But patients who receive what they consider good spiritual care feel more contented and hopeful, and have less pain and other discomfort, even as their condition gets worse. They also are more likely to enroll in hospice, where miracles can be redefined.

Trixie Dempsey, a high school teacher with three grown kids, learned this powerfully twenty-five years ago, when her sister died. Trixie is still awed by the wonder of that time, if a bit sheepish. "If I were listening to this story I'd say, yeah, what was Trixie drinking when she went into that room?" Yet she glowed when she told the story. "I think about Dottie every day."

Trixie and Dottie came from a close family that worked together in a weaving business in Yonkers, New York. Dottie, a former nun, had a baby girl at the age of forty-one, and two months later started having back pain. By the time she was diagnosed with breast cancer, it had spread everywhere. Nine months of treatment left her unable to sit up, her back broken in four places. The doctor prescribed pills for the pain even though she could not swallow.

A friend put them in touch with hospice, and the whole scene changed. Hospice workers came in and asked: How can I help you? "They don't make you feel stupid," Trixie said. "They let you have your emotions. They don't ridicule them. They don't minimize them." Dottie had fought hard to

245

hang on — she wanted desperately to live, to raise her child. But once she accepted hospice, a calm came over her. She prayed with her family, reminisced, and planned her funeral and her daughter's future. "It's a very special time when you leave your life," Trixie said. Somehow, hospice made it OK.

A nurse's aide came, and when she finished washing Dottie, turning her, and doing all the other labors, the woman did not race out the door. Instead, she sat beside Dottie and sang hymns in a gorgeous soprano. "I still remember Marian and what she was wearing and where she stood and how she held Dottie's hand," Trixie said.

Marian sang "On Eagle's Wings." "We were transfixed. That somebody would do that for someone else, in such an unpretentious, unselfconscious way, just to give this hymn to Dottie, who always sang glee club in high school. She was always singing something. And then for Marian to come in . . . It was something else.

"You could see — very subtly, you'd have to really watch her — but you could see that Dottie could hear. And it was quite a beautiful, magical moment. You feel like you know that she's in a better place."

When the priest came to perform last

rites, Dottie looked up and opened her arms despite her broken back. She said, "Jesus my Lord." The priest did not look surprised.

Dottie died at five in the afternoon, nine months after she was diagnosed and two weeks before her daughter's first birthday. "And right as she took her last breath, a wind kicked up," Trixie said. "It was October, and the trees and the wind all rustled. And she was gone."

A year later, as Trixie's father was dying of colon cancer in a hospital, she knew just what to do. She, her brother, and another sister shut the door to his room, wedging in a chair to make sure they had privacy. They talked to their father as if he could hear, unembarrassed to say what they felt. Then they prayed.

CHAPTER ELEVEN:
NEW COURSE FOR DOCTORS

"This is medicine the way
I wanted to practice it."

Doctors are exquisitely trained, not to pray for us, but to make us better. So how can they help patients when a cure is not the goal? A young doctor named Thuy Nguyen struggled with the question one morning in the spring of 2011. He was completing a yearlong fellowship at San Diego Hospice and the Institute of Palliative Medicine, at the time one of the largest programs for advanced training in the field. Soon he would join a community medical practice. Now he was telling one of his mentors, Elizabeth Menkin, about a case that troubled him.

It involved an elderly woman in a nursing home who had a long list of ailments, including diabetes. She seemed to grow frailer by the day, more detached from life, until one day she announced that she wanted to die. Her grown children pleaded with her to get psychiatric help, and to please them, she agreed. It did not change her mind, only made her more determined. She stopped taking her insulin, knowing it would kill her, and she asked for a hospice referral. Nguyen got the call.

Every first-year medical student learns about the complications of untreated diabetes, called DKA, or diabetes ketoacidosis. Acid builds up in the blood, and the metabolism goes haywire, causing dehydration, severe disorientation, and death. Medical students also learn to treat the condition by administering insulin, fluids, and electrolytes. Allowing it to run its fatal course is not in the manual or in the realm of possibility. As Nguyen told Menkin, "I'm not used to letting people die of DKA."

But that's what his patient wanted, and that's what he did. He arranged for intensive support from the hospice team. He had drugs at the ready in case of pain. He talked at length with the woman and her family. When her children asked what would happen as her body shut down, he told them he had never seen anyone die of her condition.

Around day three without insulin, she

took to her bed for the last time. The next day, she developed some delirium — confusion and incoherence caused by chemical changes in the brain. This happens commonly at the very end of life, and it can distress patients, so he prescribed a benzodiazepine, which helped. On the tenth day, she died peacefully, yet somehow he felt he should have done more.

Menkin saw no red flags or missteps. She reminded Nguyen that a patient with decision-making capacity has the right to refuse even a standard treatment like insulin. Of course, he knew this. But on some level a doctor is like a dancer with muscle memory, and his muscles had been chiseled by four years of medical school and four years of residency training in a hospital. True, he had just spent the year training in palliative medicine, acquiring the knowledge and skills to relieve suffering without trying to forestall death. Still, his doctor's instincts insisted that truly helping patients means curing them.

Sometimes, he told Menkin, he went to nursing homes to check up on hospice patients who had so many serious conditions that it wasn't clear which one would kill them, and he felt useless: "I don't know what to do for them."

So she ran down a list: Be present. Listen to their stories. Bear witness to their courage. Keep them comfortable. Honor their wishes. Don't impose yours. "Hospice isn't about taking care of diseases," she said. "You're taking care of people."

Why Relief of Suffering Should Be Standard Medical Practice

As of May 2012, eighty-five fellowship programs in hospice and palliative medicine trained hundreds of doctors each year in the science and art of symptom management and comfort. Most of these physicians will spend their careers not in hospice but in family medicine, internal medicine, pediatrics, oncology, emergency medicine, surgery, cardiology, psychiatry, and other specialties. That is the point. For too long, relieving suffering was the exclusive purview of one specialty, palliative medicine, available only in a niche called hospice. In other words, people had to be near death and on hospice to see professionals who were highly trained to manage physical, emotional, and spiritual suffering. To say that made no sense is an understatement. Most Americans still die in hospitals, despite the rapid growth of hospice. They should have access to the best that modern medicine offers, including palliative care. Nor are pain and suffering limited to patients on the brink of death. If we were to stop and think about it, most of us would want any doctor who might treat us for cancer, heart disease, diabetes, or any other serious problem to possess the skills and compassion to care for *us,* in addition to caring for our illness.

In 1996, a psychologist painted such a dismal picture of end-of-life care in hospitals that it seemed as if Elisabeth Kübler-Ross and Cicely Saunders had never been born. "A thin veneer of physician arrogance cannot eclipse the truth of most Americans' last days," she wrote in a letter to the *New York Times.* "Physicians almost uniformly avoid, ignore, and panic when faced with terminally ill patients. It has been my displeasure to have a keenly sensitive woman realize how short her time on this earth would be, based on how quickly her oncologist evaporated from the examining room."

That same year, only six of the nation's 126 medical schools required courses in end-of-life care. Nursing schools did no better. A 1999 analysis of fifty major nursing education textbooks, totaling 45,683 pages, found that only 2 percent of those pages seriously addressed symptom assessment and management at the end of life.

Today medical schools must provide such instruction in order to be accredited, though each can determine what it teaches and how. Until the early 2000s, students at the University of Pittsburgh School of Medicine would receive three hours of formal instruction on end-of-life issues during their first two years. Students would learn more if they opted to work with terminally ill patients during the latter part of medical school. Few did, which is not surprising. When a topic receives such cursory treatment, students get the message about where it ranks on the value scale (not to mention the pay scale) of medicine.

Beginning with the class of 2006, the school integrated content on end-of-life care into the coursework of the first two years, and students learned about it not only from their professors but also from patients and families. Many other medical schools also do a better job of incorporating the topic into the curriculum and bringing students face-to-face with patients. Some medical schools send students on home visits with hospice physicians. This can be revelatory, especially because, in their personal lives, young doctors do not have much experience with death. A study by researchers at Stanford University found that only 6 percent of interns (first-year doctors, training in hospitals) had experienced the death of a close relative.

During their hospital training they will see plenty of people die, almost always in emergency rooms and intensive care units after frantic measures fail to staunch catastrophic bleeding or restart the heart. Yet most lives do not end so quickly or violently but slowly, bit by agonizing bit. "While interns had cared for many patients who died," the researchers wrote, "they had learned little about dying."

Many new doctors acknowledge this, at least in anonymous surveys. In a 2012 questionnaire by the Association of American Medical Colleges, nearly one in five graduating medical students rated their instruction in palliative care and pain management as inadequate. One in six gave the same failing grade to their instruction on end-of-life issues, such as removing life supports or talking with patients about hospice.

Young doctors have time to learn, of course. Medical school graduation leads straight into years of hospital-based internship and residency. That is the boot camp, drilling doctors day in and day out on the methods and mores of their profession.

"What students hear in medical school has no effect on their practice whatsoever," said Charles F. von Gunten, editor in chief of the *Journal of Palliative Medicine*. "You really learn to be a doctor in residency, so the most important influence on how a doctor turns out is the culture in the training hospital."

Training hospitals have come a long way in incorporating palliative techniques and addressing end-of-life care. As a resident in internal medicine in the early 1970s, Elizabeth Menkin learned nothing about any of it. In 1997, the American Board of Internal Medicine made end-of-life instruction an education requirement for residents (although, as a report by the Robert Wood Johnson Foundation noted, the senior physicians who served as mentors had little training in providing end-of-life care or in teaching the subject). In 2008, the board administered its first exam to certify hospice and palliative medicine as a subspecialty. In 2012, 70 percent of the nation's 400 major teaching hospitals had a palliative medicine service. This incorporates a hospice-style approach — interdisciplinary, holistic, focused on symptom control — into acute care, to help patients who have serious or chronic illnesses but who are not necessarily near death.

In the public mind, there is confusion between hospice and palliative care. Patients sometimes panic and even become angry when they are referred for a palliative consult. They think it means hospice or "death panels," or that their own doctors are giving up. More and more, what it means is that a trained professional — or better yet, an interdisciplinary team — will focus on helping the person feel better while he or she tries to get better. Many people also think, wrongly, that if they accept palliative services they will have to stop curative treatments, as Medicare and most other insurers effectively force hospice patients to do. Because palliative care is relatively new, insurance coverage is evolving, but Medicare, Medicaid, and private plans do not require people to choose between standard medical treatments and the comforts offered by a palliative care service.

The growth of palliative medicine reflects a long-overdue recognition that the health care system fails patients by waiting until they are about to die before addressing the pain and anguish brought on (or to the surface) by their illness and its arduous treatments. A woman with stage 2 breast cancer, for instance, may have great survival odds, but the surgery, chemotherapy, and radiation she must endure over months will have brutal side effects. In addition to all that great cancer treatment, why not call in professionals to provide effective relief for nausea, nerve pain, or awful skin burns? Why not offer this woman and millions of others the benefit of palliative expertise honed over decades in hospices, instead of holding off until the disease is too advanced to turn back?

These questions have gained urgency in the wake of research suggesting that early palliative care does more than provide desperately needed relief. It also extends lives. In a three-year study of 151 patients with terminal lung cancer, those who received palliative care combined with standard oncology treatment upon diagnosis experienced less pain and nausea, felt happier, and were more mobile as the end approached than patients who received only standard cancer treatment. And the palliative group lived nearly three months longer. The survival benefit was especially striking because far fewer patients in the palliative group chose aggressive chemotherapy as their illness progressed, and more signed orders not to be revived if their heart or breathing stopped.

The study involved only a small group of patients and one type of cancer. Nevertheless, the American Society of Clinical oncology considered the findings so compelling that, just months after they were published, the group issued a provisional recommendation that palliative care be incorporated into standard cancer oncology practice as soon as anyone is diagnosed with cancer that has spread.

Patients and families are not the only ones who stand to gain. When hospitals and clinics add palliative care to their menu of services, doctors learn what it means, see it in action, and get the message that it is integral to modern medicine — not some touchy-feely approach reserved for hospice.

That is the hope, anyway. We are not there yet. Academic medical centers represent only 7 percent of all hospitals in the United States. Palliative care has yet to filter down to thousands of community hospitals. And even at some — perhaps many — teaching hospitals with busy, well-regarded palliative care services, old habits and biases hold firm.

"Some of our older mentors do not want to talk about palliative care," said Lauren Van Scoy, a physician who was about to complete advanced training in pulmonary and critical care medicine in Philadelphia. "I know an oncologist who refuses to have palliative care for any of her patients."

Van Scoy gets more done in a week than most of us accomplish in a year. She worked a breakneck schedule in the intensive care unit. After watching so many patients and families struggle to make health care decisions in the heat of a crisis, she developed a tool, the Last Wish Compass, to help them plan in advance. It leads people, step by step, through complex health care choices. She also wrote poignant stories about patients in the ICU and published them, along with the tool, in a book: *Last Wish: Stories to Inspire a Peaceful Passing.*

The ICU is not typically a place where people talk about peaceful endings. How did her colleagues react?

"If you were to ask them formally they'd say, oh, it's so important. But they tease: 'What are you doing working in the ICU if you just want to have end-of-life conversations?' " Van Scoy said. "My field can be a boys' club. Sometimes it feels like your value is in how much you do in a night. How many intubations did you do? How much blood did you get on yourself during call last night? They see me, and because I also have interests in things besides aggressive interventions in the ICU, like family meetings and counseling about end of life, they may tease, 'Oooh, here comes Dr. Death.'"

The United States has 850,000 licensed physicians, and we are all fortunate that some of them chose the work because they love the adrenaline rush of emergencies and rescue. And we are lucky that others chose it because they love cutting people open to repair a heart or remove a malignant tumor, or because they are fascinated by the intricacies of treating cancer, diabetes, and other conditions that once were fatal. Yet we are also fortunate that more and more doctors think about healing, not just curing, and that they measure their professional worth not by the number of tubes they insert but by the depth of their connections with patients.

For doctors like this, training in hospice and palliative care, even for a brief stint, can be transformative. "Uniformly it's, 'Aah, this reminds me of why I wanted to be a doctor,'" von Gunten said. "It has nothing to do with end-of-life care. It's, 'This is medicine the way I wanted to practice it. This is health care the way it should be done. Why is this not the way we treat patients in the hospital across the street?' "

From Diet Pills to Dying Patients

Elizabeth Menkin always wanted to be a doctor. She worked for years as an internist at Kaiser Permanente, one of the nation's oldest and largest nonprofit integrated health systems — first in Santa Clara, California, and then in neighboring San Jose. Diet pills, of all things, pushed her into geriatrics, which in turn led her to hospice. "Fen-phen and what was the other hot one? They hit the front of *Newsweek*," she recalled. "People would come in and they'd want me to write a prescription. And I was like, yeah, you think maybe you could take in fewer calories? And they were, 'oh I've got this cellulite, I've got to do something about this cellulite, I don't eat that much!' And it was all I could do not to say, gee that's funny, nobody left Auschwitz with cellulite except the guards."

She took that as a sign that she needed a change of scene. She started working in nursing homes and loved it that people there "don't sweat the small stuff." Menkin never looked back. "After about six months, I thought, this is really great. Nobody's asked me for diet pills. They've asked me for a lot of other things but nobody has asked me for diet pills. I had this sense that in the outpatient clinic I could go weeks without seeing someone who really needed a doctor. But so many times, I felt the nursing home patients and their families really need somebody with the skills I have for symptom management, health education, and counseling."

Working with hospice patients and families offered the same gratification. "Even when I can't make things better, I can at least bear witness to what they're going through and normalize it. Tell them it's not their fault. This is the way it feels. Some days Mom is clear and some days she's not — that's typical at this stage. It feels like a roller coaster. This is normal — it's unusual for a patient to have a nice steady slope where you can predict what tomorrow will look like based on the changes from yesterday until today."

When Menkin turned sixty, in 2008, she took early retirement, bought a condo 420 miles south, and went to work at the nonprofit San Diego Hospice and Institute of Palliative Medicine. It was one of the largest academic hospices in the world and widely regarded as an innovator. It cared for about a thousand patients a day, operated a state-of-the-art twenty-four-bed inpatient facility, trained hundreds of doctors from all over the world, and pushed the bounds of hospice care — for example, through pioneering work in palliative psychiatry and aromatherapy.

Menkin's move had some personal downsides. Her husband, Bill, an elementary school teacher, had to stay in San Jose, leaving them to commute. But she could not pass up the opportunity to train a new generation of doctors or join a program renowned for its expansive view of hospice.

Soon after her arrival, Menkin took part in a group exercise that had thirty-five doctors, from fellows to senior staff, spend five minutes scribbling answers to the question, "What keeps you in palliative medicine?" Almost nobody wrote a word about science, technology, or even medicine. Instead, they wrote:

"The opportunity to make changes, no matter how small, for people who are suffering."

"Valuing relationships with patients, among family members."

"The openness to new thoughts and ideas."

When a Patient Is Ready to Go Home

House calls are an old idea, a throwback to the days when families had a Dr. Welby to call upon, day or night. They are a mainstay of hospice care. When Elizabeth Menkin walks into houses, people often treat her like a dignitary. It's a safe bet that almost none of them has had a doctor ring their doorbell in a half-century, if ever. Nurses and aides do most of the hospice home visits, but unless a patient dies right after enrolling, a doctor typically will come, assess his or her condition, and answer the family's questions.

One morning, Menkin visited a small rectangle of a house that looked like every other on its suburban street. The patient, in her eighties, had mild dementia, heart problems, and kidney failure diagnosed just a few days earlier, while she was hospitalized for chest pain. She refused dialysis, signed up for hospice, and returned to the house she had moved into as a young bride. She sat in a dark brown leather recliner in the living room, feet up. A hand-crocheted blanket covered her from tummy to toes. She tried to stand in greeting when the doctor entered. Menkin smiled and motioned her to stay seated. The woman thanked Menkin twice for coming, and her husband offered to make tea.

"How are you feeling?" Menkin asked the woman.

"Pretty good."

Menkin asked her permission to lift and look underneath the blanket. She palpated the belly gently, ran her hands and her eyes along the legs, removed the baby blue fuzzy socks on the feet, and remarked on the swelling from water retention, common in kidney failure.

Menkin lowered the foot into her lap but kept holding it and looked the woman in the eye.

"I'm ready," the woman said. "I'm ready to go home."

"You are home," her husband said from across the room.

She paid him no attention. "I'm satisfied. I'm ready," she repeated.

"That's a good feeling," Menkin said. She spoke naturally, not loudly or r-e-a-l-l-y s-l-o-w-l-y, as people often do with seniors and little kids. "What about your family? Are they ready?"

The husband leaned wearily in the doorway. "When we brought her home, the doctors said it would be days. Days? Is that two days? Six days? Thirty?"

Menkin said it generally means a week for patients who stop dialysis. It's harder to predict for someone like his wife, who never had dialysis.

"I'm ready," the woman repeated.

"Sometimes she has delusions," her husband told Menkin. "The other night she saw termites marching up the wall."

Was she having a delusion now? Did the unlikely presence of a doctor in her home confuse her, make her think she was back in the hospital, where she had made it plain she did not want to stay?

Or did this woman know what was happening, and did she mean exactly what everyone assumed?

Back in the office that afternoon, Menkin would say she had heard countless geriatric patients say they were ready to die. "And it doesn't correlate with life being lousy. It's like when kids are at a puppet show. The show's ongoing and they love it. But there comes a point — you just don't want to keep watching the show forever. I get this sense from many older patients, a sense of *been there, done that.* Sometimes people seem wistful: 'I'd like to stick around longer but I know that's not in the cards for me.' But there's no anger or grief about it."

Everyone Dies Differently

If hospice doctors (and nurses, social workers, aides, and even people who write hospice books) have one thing in common, it's the question they hear all the time: Isn't that depressing?

In fact, surveys show that doctors in palliative medicine have among the highest rates of satisfaction and lowest rates of burnout of all physicians. "Burnout happens when you're faced with meaningless work," Menkin said. "I find this very meaningful. You have the privilege of being let into people's lives at an enormously important and needy time."

That answer, it turns out, may be as common among hospice physicians as the question. "You see results quickly. You have to," said Ellen Brown, medical director at Pathways Home Health & Hospice in the San Francisco Bay Area. "I am in awe of how families come together."

This does not mean the hospice doctor finds every household harmonious or every patient awaiting the end with a beatific smile. Everyone dies differently, and while a surprising number of elderly people may tell a doctor they're ready, just as many patients, probably more, rail against fate. Elizabeth Menkin converted to Judaism years ago, and, when a workday took her from a patient at one extreme to a patient at the other, she often thought of a rabbinic tale about the deaths of Moses and his brother, Aaron.

The story begins with Moses on the mountaintop, about to die just before the Israelites cross into the Promised Land. God is punishing him for displaying a lack of faith when he struck the rock twice in the desert, instead of telling it to produce water, as God had commanded. "Moses, who's famously tongue-tied, is arguing with God," Menkin said. " 'Why do I have to go? It's kind of a harsh sentence. Yeah, I was supposed to talk to the rock, and I hit the rock, but is that a capital crime? I served you this long, can't I have an extension on this job?' Argue, argue, argue, until finally, God has to take Moses's breath and his soul with a kiss, draw his breath out of him, to stop the argument."

Aaron, known for his eloquence, also dies in the desert. "The description is that his priestly garments are folded up and delivered to his son," Menkin said. "And he lies down and dies — very compliant, nice closure, nice transition to the next generation. No fighting and digging in his heels. These are brothers!

"Some people die like Moses, and some people die like Aaron. It's not to say that one's right and one's wrong. And it's not to say you could predict that the one who was tongue-tied is going to be arguing until the last breath, and the one who was the speaker will be silent. Sometimes I just have to remind myself that some people are going to die like Moses and some people are going to die like Aaron."

Breaking Bad News

One afternoon, Menkin gathered eight third-year medical students into a circle. It was their first of four required visits to a hospice, and they began with an hour-long workshop on breaking bad news. A professional actress entered, playing the role of Alexa Bailey, a forty-seven-year-old wife, mother, and breast cancer patient who had come to the doctor to get the results of a recent bone scan. Her skin looked wan. A scarf covered what was presumably her bald skull. But Alexa smiled and had a slight spring in her step.

She announced she was feeling stronger these days, and she knew, just knew, that meant the latest chemo regimen was working. One by one, the students took turns playing the doctor who had to say no, the scans looked bad, she would not get better, she might want to consider hospice. Menkin explained that she would call "stop" to break for a teachable moment, hear a student's thought, or put the next student in the hot seat. She would call "rewind" when a student said something that he or she should rethink and rephrase.

The exercise began. By turns, the students spoke of "metastases" and cancer "progressing." Alexa looked perplexed, then tearful. She asked one "doctor" after another, What are you saying? Her voice grew pinched, more frantic each time she repeated the question, until she started sobbing. Most eyes in the circle welled up. But nobody came out with it straight and uttered the *d*-word. Finally, she pleaded, "Does this mean I am going to die?"

In every molded plastic chair, a body stiffened. After a beat of silence, the student in the hot seat spoke. "There's nothing we can do about it."

Rewind.

"Well, we have gotten to a point where more chemo will not stop the cancer."

Stop.

Released from the doctor role, the student said, "I think I was as nervous as she was," and then burst out crying. "I'm sorry. I have no idea why I'm so upset. I think it's easier in real life. I have my white coat. I know what's expected."

But did she? As the hour ended, the

students reflected on what happened. "Very tough, very tough, very tough conversation to have," one said. Another said he did not want to make the patient feel as if he were "giving up" on her, and many heads nodded. A student wondered whether they had all stumbled around because they did not want to take away her hope.

What hope can they offer? Like these students and like the young doctor Thuy Nguyen, physicians have wrestled with this question since the earliest days of hospice. In his 1996 essay "The Doctor's Role in Death," Yale surgeon Sherwin B. Nuland pointed out that hope is connected to the future, and hopelessness in essence means that a person believes his or her future is lost. Isn't that also the essence of dying — the future stripped away?

Not necessarily. "One does not need to believe in an afterlife to believe there is a future for those who are dying, and hope in visualizing that future," Nuland wrote. "As I look over definitions of hope, I find many meanings but only one universal: hope lies in the expectation of a good that is yet to be." The last months, even the final days, can provide some of the most indelible moments in life.

■ ■ ■ ■

In a perfect world, a chapter on hospice doctors would end right there. But hospice doctors must master another skill, one that has nothing to do with caring for patients or talking with families. Just as Florence Wald, the founder of hospice in the United States, saw her high ideals squeezed by economic and political pressures, today's hospice doctors and nurses often complain that Medicare rules compromise best practices. Hospices are under orders to hold down costs and document every move. This is happening throughout health care, but the pressures have increased on hospice especially because a lot of money is at stake. Fewer and fewer hospices operate as charitable enterprises anymore. Hospice has become big business.

CHAPTER TWELVE:
DYING FOR DOLLARS

"Even I am surprised at the amount of money waiting to come in — three billion dollars . . . looking for entry points to the hospice world."

From a mission of mercy, hospice has evolved into a $14 billion industry, increasingly run by corporate chains, and nobody gets more credit, or blame, than the Reverend Hugh Westbrook. He invented the very idea of the corporate hospice, when he and a couple of partners opened the first for-profit program, in Dallas, in 1984 — right after the Medicare law he was instrumental in crafting began to pay for hospice services. Over the next two decades, he grew the company into VITAS Innovative Hospice Care, the largest hospice chain in the United States — or anywhere, for that matter, because hospice chains do not exist abroad. In the process, Westbrook proved the unthinkable: A business can make a fortune caring for dying people.

Certainly he did. He had yachts, a Florida beachfront mansion, and a mountain home in North Carolina. He invested in a string of companies. He wrote big checks to Democratic candidates — his name would turn up on an infamous list of donors who received an invitation to sleep in the White House Lincoln Bedroom in exchange for a minimum $50,000 donation to President Clinton's re-election campaign. And all that happened before he made the really big money, by cashing out to Roto-Rooter, a publicly traded company and a longtime VITAS investor.

Roto-Rooter already owned about 25 percent of VITAS when it acquired the rest of the company, in a $406 million deal in 2004. Westbrook walked away with about $200 million.

He signed the standard agreements not to compete, which kept him out of the hospice world for eight years. In that time, the industry changed more dramatically than even he could have imagined. A wave of mergers, acquisitions, and investments made hospice another Wall Street commodity to be traded, with one goal: maximizing returns. Roto-Rooter kept its hospice operations under the VITAS name but rebranded the corporate parent as Chemed Corp. The name had a ring of scientific authority and did not call to mind clogged drains.

Now under pressure to please shareholders with ever-larger revenues each quarter, VITAS embarked on a fast track to growth. It bought smaller hospices, opened new ones, and marketed more aggressively to doctors — for example, the free VITAS app, released in 2012, offered doctors the convenience of making referrals "without ever leaving your phone." The company also began advertising directly to consumers, on radio and billboards. In 2012, VITAS had 11,000 employees in fifty-one programs across eighteen states. It served more than 75,000 patients and reported nearly $1 billion in revenues. As VITAS supersized, salaries bulked up too, at least in the corner offices of the corporate suite. Kevin J. McNamara, Chemed president and CEO, earned $6.4 million in salary, bonuses, stock awards, and other compensation in 2011. Timothy S. O'Toole, head of the VITAS subsidiary, had a $2.7 million package.

No wonder hospice beckoned investors. Almost every hospice program opened in the past decade has been for-profit. By 2011, 60 percent of Medicare-certified hospice providers were for-profit companies, up from 27 percent ten years earlier. Gentiva Health Services Inc., a publicly traded home health company, bought up small hospice chains in an aggressive move into the hospice market. (Yes, people in end-of-life care, at for-profits and nonprofits alike, now toss around phrases like "the hospice market." In investor circles, it's "the hospice space.") By 2012, Gentiva operated hospice programs in 165 locations across thirty states, with net revenues of $765 million.

While such numbers pointed to a dizzying pace of consolidation in a field that had always prided itself on local autonomy and deep community roots, these two hospice giants, together, accounted for less than 15 percent of all spending for hospice care. That left a lot of tantalizing territory wide open. Venture capital and private equity firms began staking their claims. The first three months of 2011 logged ten big equity investments in hospice companies, a near record. "Hospice deal volume continues to roll," proclaimed *Becker's Hospital Review*, a health care business journal, as it named hospice one of "thirteen hot areas for private equity investment." (*Becker's* placed home health care on its "cold" list, which might explain Gentiva's push into hospice.)

A typical newcomer was Sentinel Capital Partners, a Manhattan-based equity firm with a mission "to generate attractive investment returns." In 2012, Sentinel added Hospice Advantage, a chain with fifty-six programs across the Midwest and the South, to a diverse portfolio of companies, including Huddle House family restaurants; Trussbilt LLC, a manufacturer of steel doors for prisons; Spinrite, a yarn maker; and National Spine & Pain Centers. The financially beleaguered Washington Post Co. also came on the scene, acquiring a majority stake in Celtic Healthcare, a Pennsylvania-based home health and home hospice provider. In a statement quoted in his own newspaper, Chief Executive Donald Graham — an heir to a proud legacy of journalism in the public trust — said the deal was "part of the Post Company's ongoing strategy of investing in companies with demonstrated earnings potential." In 2013, the Washington Post Co. sold the newspaper, but kept the hospice holdings.

The commercialization of hospice generated less enthusiasm outside the investment community. As the market heated up, hospice attracted the worst publicity in its history, dimming its halo image, fairly or not. The U.S. Department of Justice sued several hospices for milking, or bilking, Medicare for millions of dollars — in some cases by enrolling elderly patients who were not terminally ill. A blistering investigation by Bloomberg reporter Peter Waldman uncovered sales contests and high-pressure marketing tactics at a few for-profits — including a "Christmas Cash Blitz," a "Fall Frenzy," and a "September Sizzle" at a hospice in Kansas that paid employees as much as $100 a head for referrals. On the clinical side, a long-time hospice nurse, Nancy Costea, published a powerful essay in the journal *Nursing Forum* in which she chronicled the harried pace of her job, the large caseloads, and the fragmentation of care that left patients in the hands of a parade of unfamiliar nurses and aides, eroding the intimate bond between health care provider and patient that once defined hospice care.

Costea worked for VistaCare Hospice in Albuquerque, a small, well-regarded chain founded in 1995 by three nurses and a health care entrepreneur. A larger chain, Odyssey HealthCare, acquired VistaCare in 2008 for $147 million. Two years later, Gentiva bought Odyssey for nearly $1 billion. Costea's account eerily echoed the criticisms that Elisabeth Kübler-Ross and Florence Wald had leveled at hospitals decades before — the frenzied, impersonal conditions that gave rise to the hospice alternative in the first place. Costea wrote of her struggle to do her job without losing her "hospice heart," giving public voice to a sentiment that more and more nurses and doctors expressed among themselves. Over coffee or a glass of wine at the end of a long day, they would talk about the bureaucracy, the marketers, and ask, often with a guilty grimace: Was hospice in danger of losing its soul?

Hugh Westbrook, of all people, wondered too.

He re-emerged on the hospice scene in 2012, freed from the contract that had sidelined him. "About two and a half seconds after my non-compete agreement expired I started getting calls from private equity firms saying, 'Are you ready to go and build another company' and 'We really want to get into this,' " he recently said. "Even I am surprised at the amount of money waiting to come in — three billion dollars of venture capital and private equity money looking for entry points to the hospice world."

Westbrook explored several opportunities, reviewed business plans, studied earnings projections. He saw investor groups eyeing hospices not as he did — "it's my life's work" — but strictly for short-term gains: "Programs have been started so they can run for a year and be sold, so somebody can make money flipping them and go to the next place and start again." In the end, he turned down the deals that came his way. He worried about the dark side of private equity, with its single-minded focus on the bottom line. He did not want to see hospice become just another target for corporate raiders, a property to be purchased, stripped, and sold at a handsome profit.

"I don't think the entrance of venture capital and private equity into the hospice world in a very aggressive way is good for what hospice is about and tries to do," he said. "I think it's a threat."

Westbrook recognized the irony in his stance. Many people considered him a threat and a sellout when he took the first step down the for-profit path. But whether you admire or loathe what he did and where it led, there was no denying that he set out to make a difference for patients, not to make a quick buck off them.

"I'm sure this is not apparent to you," he said, "but we really believed in what we were doing."

■ ■ ■ ■

From the day Hugh Westbrook founded his company with Esther Colliflower, a nurse, and Donald Gaetz, a health care executive, the hospice world has wrestled with a question: Do for-profits provide good patient care, or do they cut corners to increase their margins? Hospices that receive Medicare money — and more than 90 percent do — are required to offer core services, including nursing, physician oversight, social support, spiritual care, bereavement support, and home-delivered medications, supplies, and equipment. This sets the bar fairly high for all programs, nonprofits and for-profits alike.

"I never saw care diminished," said Jamie Floyd, a social worker who worked as the national director of marketing and education of the Odyssey chain before leaving the hospice industry. "It's so regulated, and you have so much to lose."

But hospices have leeway in determining how to fulfill some of these mandates, and they do not have go beyond the requirements. One hospice may have a spiritual care program staffed by ordained clergy of all faiths certified in clinical pastoral education. Another may rely on volunteers from a local church who stop by the bedside and pray when a patient requests it. One hospice may proactively screen family caregivers for signs of depression or debilitating grief and run specialty bereavement groups for the loss of a spouse, of a parent, of a child. Another hospice may check up on survivors now and then by phone — that's the bereavement program. One hospice may offer massage therapy or music therapy, or dispatch a psychotherapist to talk with patients about the kind of legacy they would like to leave. Others do no such thing because Medicare does not require or pay for it.

There is no research evidence that for-profits provide lower-quality care than non-profits, or higher-quality. But they have lower costs (which gives them higher margins) for a few reasons that can have a significant effect on a patient's experience. For one, for-profits on average employ less-skilled staff at the bedside. A study of 3,927 hospices, published in the *Journal of Palliative Medicine* in 2010, found that for-profits have proportionally fewer high-end professionals such as registered nurses and medical social workers — the sort of trained, educated staff "prepared to care for patients with terminal illnesses and their families," the researchers wrote.

Second, for-profits tend to admit the most lucrative patients. Hospices are paid a flat daily rate for each patient, regardless of the diagnosis — Medicare paid an average $157 a day in 2012 for routine home care. But a hospice's costs to care for that patient fluctuate. Patients and families need the most attention (and staff time) in the first three to seven days and again in the final days before death, so the costs run highest then. Between those end points, the patient's condition and the family's situation often stabilize. Nurses and social workers have to visit less frequently. Doctors and pharmacists have to respond to fewer emergency calls. If things are going well, the hospice may have no direct contact at all with the family on a given day, yet the hospice still collects that $157. The payment formula means that hospices can lose money on the patient who dies soon after enrolling. They make the most money on the patient they hang on to for the longest time.

Such patients turn out to be the for-profit sweet spot. A study of 1,036 hospice agencies, published in the *Journal of the American Medical Association* in 2011, found that for-profits have far more patients who stay six months, a year, even longer. Some for-profits actively recruit patients who have dementia and other illnesses that progress slowly and often unpredictably — people who might fit the Medicare requirement of a six-month life expectancy, yet who may linger well beyond that. Compared with nonprofits, for-profits, on average, have fewer patients with cancer — people who often need more intensive hospice support, especially to manage pain, and who tend to enroll just days or weeks before they die.

Another way to protect the bottom line is by restricting palliative treatments. In the early days of hospice, the medical management of pain pretty much meant one thing: opioids. That's still the case in many hospices, even though medical advances have opened up a world of options, especially for people with late-stage cancer. For example, palliative radiation can shrink a tumor pressing on nerves. Palliative chemotherapy has been shown to decrease pain and other symptoms of advanced pancreatic, prostate, and lung cancers. The old-line, relatively low-tech blood transfusion can strengthen a patient, helping him or her function better and enjoy life more.

None of this comes cheaply. A course of palliative radiation can run about $7,500. A unit of blood ranges from $500 to $1,200. Medicare does not require hospices to provide these treatments or pay hospices extra if they do. Some hospices — generally large independent nonprofits or university-affiliated programs — offer such treatments anyway, even without special reimbursement, when they are necessary to keep a patient comfortable. But under cost pressure from Medicare, many hospices — for-profits and nonprofits both — refuse to provide radiation, transfusions, and other services that they say cross the (increasingly fuzzy) line between palliative care and life-prolonging therapy. For-profits are much stricter on this score, and they are less likely to accept a patient who may need expensive or extensive palliative care, lest they get stuck with the bill.

What happens when such a patient ends up in a for-profit program? In the case of Michelle Hargett Beebee, nothing good. A forty-three-year-old single mother of three, Michelle was diagnosed with pancreatic cancer and enrolled in a VITAS program in late November 2009. She died in her apartment, in Los Gatos, California, after three weeks of unrelieved pain and distress.

It probably goes without saying that the family expected better. Michelle had enrolled in hospice in the hope that she would die in comfort and dignity — two soothing, alluring words on VITAS promotional material. That hope had lifted her spirits, and her family's too, after the shock and devastation of her diagnosis. The family received the referral at the county medical center, where Michelle had been hospitalized. Desperate and overwhelmed, they never thought to research whether this was the best program in the region or to question the hospital social worker about the brand. "It's like saying, 'Here's some Kleenex.' 'Oh, thanks.' You don't think, oh, which kind of Kleenex?" said Michelle's mother, Carol Hargett. "Next thing you know we're in a meeting room, we're going, 'Oh my God, she's going through so much pain. Please hurry!' "

VITAS physicians prescribed methadone every eight hours and rectal morphine for breakthrough pain. But nothing helped. Of all the torments of those weeks, the thought of her children hurt worst. "Michelle did not want her children to remember her that way," said her father, Joe Hargett. When the Hargetts called the hospice to say Michelle was in agony, Carol said, they were told that everything possible was being done. An hour before dawn on a December morning,

Michelle's screaming finally stopped, and Carol knew she was dead.

Eleven months later, Carol and Joe sued VITAS, claiming the hospice had deprived their daughter of a peaceful death. The suit charged that doctors did not treat her pain or inform her of treatment alternatives, as California law requires, and that poorly trained employees failed to relay the family's complaints to the physicians. In particular, the Hargetts asserted that the hospice should have informed them and Michelle about palliative sedation — a last-resort treatment they did not learn about until much later. It uses strong drugs to render a patient unconscious until death, when suffering is intolerable and resistant to all other measures for relief.

As of early 2013, no trial date had been set, and VITAS had lost several attempts to have large portions of the case dismissed. Palliative sedation is controversial and used only in extreme situations, but, whatever the outcome of the case, the Hargetts hoped to illuminate a human issue. "This company has 10,000 patients a day in hospice," Carol said. "We're just a number."

As it happens, volume has increased since the Hargetts first encountered VITAS. In

2012, the company served 14,000 patients a day.

The Accidental Entrepreneur

"I'm very interested in what's happening now in the hospice — well, what I still refer to as the hospice movement but is today the hospice industry," Hugh Westbrook said in his affable Southern drawl.

He may be the last person in America to still call it a movement, yet that sense of purpose brought him to Washington, D.C., on a steamy August day. He sat in a sleek conference room of a large legal firm — a room he used as his office whenever he came to town. He wore a sea-blue shirt, slightly rumpled and open at the collar. Just as he had in his Medicare lobbying days, he jotted thoughts on yellow legal pads. Today the ink flowed, because he had a big plan. He was creating Caring Foundations, a national organization to help independent community-based nonprofits survive the competitive onslaught without losing their hospice hearts, through large-scale efficiencies such as joint purchasing and administrative operations.

"I have friends who run small and medium-size programs who used to be single providers in their community, who now have seventeen or eighteen competitors and all of them are for-profit. And these are often coming into the market in inappropriate ways. 'How many doctors can we hire and get on our payroll here?' — doctors who, coincidentally, can be referring to us. 'What kind of a relationship can we have with the local nursing home?' — which, coincidentally, is going to be sliding patients into the hospice in abusive ways?" He took a swig of Diet Coke and went on: "Losing the voice of this group of community-based programs would be a bad thing. The repository of people who are driven by mission and values in the hospice world is this group."

To anyone who has followed the hospice movement, or industry, over the years, this seems a little like Darth Vader rallying his forces to help the Jedi. But say that to Westbrook, or even lift your eyebrows in a hint of surprise (or skepticism), and he will launch into his story. He will tell you how the son of a struggling Railway Express agent in Jacksonville, Florida, grew up to become a crusading minister. How that minister became an altruistic champion for hospice care. And how that champion became a wealthy hospice entrepreneur, an outcome he insists he never intended. "The fact that a lot of money was made in creating all that value was actually accidental," he said.

People in hospice reacted with outrage when Westbrook and Gaetz capitalized on the Medicare benefit they had fashioned and opened a for-profit hospice. Many hospice founders hated the idea on principle, and some felt personally betrayed. They had walked the halls of Congress alongside Westbrook and Gaetz, lobbying for the law because they believed in the mission down to their bones. They had agreed with Westbrook when he argued that Medicare coverage was the only way to professionalize and sustain the hospice enterprise. Had it all been a smokescreen so he could get rich? Some people thought so, and thirty years later it still rankled. "They had this proprietary model in mind the whole damn time," said Madalon Amenta, former executive director of the Hospice Nurses Association.

Westbrook says no, he did not conceive of a hospice company until Medicare announced its reimbursement rates. They were low — originally $45.48 a day per patient for routine home care, roughly 20 percent less than he spent to care for patients in the two nonprofit Florida hospice programs he operated. (Many hospice administrators complained about the rates, but most programs at the time were not qualified to meet the government's standards for staffing and services; when Medicare began certifying hospices for reimbursement, fewer than 10 percent applied.) Westbrook had no background in business. He did not even know how to use a simple computer spreadsheet. But he sat down with a sixty-column accountant's pad, ran the numbers, and reached a fateful conclusion: "Hospice can't survive with this kind of reimbursement unless it really has scale."

He invited several nonprofits to team up and jointly negotiate price discounts on drugs, supplies, and equipment. The idea — reincarnated in his latest venture, Caring Foundations — went nowhere in a world of organizations run by volunteer boards of directors who felt fiercely protective of the local identity of their programs and thought it unseemly to talk about money in the same breath as hospice. He applied for bank loans but nobody wanted to finance a scrappy nonprofit. "At that point we said, let's go look for investment money." He secured his first outside investment, $3.5 million, from a large home health firm in late 1983. "And we were off."

The company grew steadily through classic business strategies: cost controls, volume purchasing, efficiencies that come with size, and marketing. The company developed the first online billing system for hospice, which sped up the notoriously slow payments from Medicare, doing wonders for cash flow. Westbrook hired marketing representatives, a job title that did not previously exist in hospice, to persuade doctors, hospitals, and nursing homes to make referrals. As he expanded his geographic reach, he committed $1 million to branding, a sum and a concept unheard of in hospice.

VITAS had a flash of embarrassing publicity on the road to riches. A 1993 investigation by the *Miami New Times,* an alternative weekly, revealed an audit showing that Westbrook had collected more than $360,000 over two years by leasing his fifty-six-foot sport fishing yacht to the company for meetings and entertainment. But nobody seriously questioned the quality of patient care. Esther Colliflower, the founder who, as a nurse, focused on the clinical side, organized care around coordinated, interdisciplinary teams. Everyone involved in a case — including volunteers, family members, and patients themselves — was invited to attend meetings and have a voice in decisions. She recently said that eliminating the fragmentation and duplication that are so common in the health care system resulted both in better care for patients and lower costs for the company.

VITAS gave away millions of dollars in charitable care and funded physician training and hospice research at universities. (VITAS and Gentiva still operate large philanthropic foundations, but for-profit hospices on the whole fall short when it comes to caring for uninsured patients.) VITAS also reached out to low-income patients and patients of color, populations that a movement born and raised in white, upper-middle-class communities overlooked shamefully for decades. "It was one of the reasons we would choose to go into a certain market — for example, into Philadelphia," Westbrook said. "No one was serving that market — mainly Medicaid, mainly African American. So we said, let's go. It's a business opportunity, besides being the right thing."

For a dozen years, VITAS faced almost no corporate competition. Then VistaCare came along, followed by Odyssey in 1996. Founded by a former VITAS sales executive, Richard Burnham, Odyssey triggered the hospice growth race, expanding fast through a buying spree. In 2000, the company turned a profit for the first time and a year later it went public. The stock offering raised $54 million, an eye-popping sum in a down year for the markets. Why such excitement for a newcomer to end-of-life care? "Investors like the large under-serviced market we are targeting," Burnham told CBS *MarketWatch*.

VITAS had brought in several large outside investors over the years, and Westbrook had always found ways to diminish their influence or buy them out so he retained control. Chemed was his sole large outside investor in 2001, and he was working on a deal to acquire its shares when Odyssey went public. "Then the marketplace got all lathered up about hospice, including Chemed. So Chemed came in and said, here's what we'll pay you for the company. It was serious multiples more than anyone had ever done."

It was, as they say, an offer he could not refuse.

As Corporate Profits Grow, So Does Medicare Spending

Since Wall Street discovered hospice, Medicare spending for hospice has shot up, from $2.9 billion in 2000 to $13 billion in 2010.

And the fastest growing population in hospice care was that most lucrative group — Alzheimer's and dementia patients, most of them living in nursing homes. From 1998 to 2008, hospice use by Alzheimer's and dementia patients increased six-fold. Hundreds of hospices, mostly for-profits, have two-thirds or more of their patients in nursing homes.

To a degree, greater hospice use by dementia patients signals progress. A nursing home patient with advanced dementia who is not on hospice will often be rushed to a hospital and resuscitated in a medical crisis, even if the family has signed a "do not resuscitate" order. If you were in a nursing home, too incapacitated to lift your head, lick food off a spoon, and remember your own name, would you want a feeding tube shoved down your throat or doctors trying to restart your heart to extend your time on earth? Or would you want hospice on call, ready to keep you comfortable and leave the rest alone?

On the other hand, it is hard to imagine a group more vulnerable to unscrupulous hospice operators than dementia patients. Abuses happen, more often though not only in the for-profit sector. In 2012 alone, Harmony Care Hospice, a small chain based in South Carolina, agreed to pay $1.3 million to settle charges that it had falsely billed Medicare for patients who were not terminally ill. Hospice Care of Kansas and its parent, Texas-based Voyager Hospice-Care, settled similar charges, for $6.1 million. Odyssey did too, in March 2012, for $25 million, in a case predating the Gentiva takeover.

The Bloomberg series detailed pushy if not odious sales practices. Hospice Care of Kansas gave salespeople a $500 monthly budget to buy meals and gifts for doctors and nursing home staff. The series opened with the story of a woman named Janet Stubbs, who had gratefully gone along with a nursing home doctor's recommendation of hospice care for her aunt. Stubbs knew the elderly woman wasn't dying, but she could not turn down free visits from a hospice nurse and a chaplain, plus an extra bath for her aunt every week — all paid by Medicare. Stubbs did not know that the hospice enrolled her aunt during its September Sizzle sales drive, which paid employees a bounty for each new customer.

With costs ballooning, the federal government is cracking down on hospices and taking a hard look at long-stay patients in non-profits and for-profits alike. In 2013, the

Office of Inspector General of the Department of Health and Human Services — the audit and investigative unit for Medicare — committed for the first time to review the marketing practices of hospices and their financial relationships with nursing homes. Signing up patients who do not belong in hospice robs taxpayers. It also violates the almost sacred trust of hospice, tainting the very word.

This does not necessarily mean that a patient on hospice care for longer than six months or a year never belonged there. The patient may have rallied under expert palliative care, an optimal outcome. Greater Medicare scrutiny is putting pressure on hospices to cut off patients who are doing really well, effectively withdrawing the very support that's keeping them alive and eroding the best traditions of hospice.

Esther Colliflower recently recalled visiting Cicely Saunders at St. Christopher's in England many years ago and seeing women lined up at the door, with small suitcases. Colliflower learned they were hospice patients who did so well under good palliative care that Saunders sent them on a few days' vacation at the beach. That ethos of helping patients to live fully — in whatever way that means to them — drove the development of hospice in this country. But it is receding ever further in today's Medicare environment. "If people are able, with proper medication, to go on trips, I see that as a success," Colliflower said. "But if it happens today, it can be looked on as fraud — 'They're well enough to go the seashore, what are they doing on hospice?' It sort of makes me bubbling mad."

The Medicare rule that eligible patients had to have a six-month life expectancy was arbitrary from the start. The government has never revised it, even though medical advances have dramatically changed the choices for people with cancer, AIDS, and other life-threatening diseases — and even though the rapidly growing population of very old patients with multiple illnesses has placed new demands on hospice providers. Predicting death is not a perfect science, especially for old people with dementia and debility.

It is not yet clear how much Medicare has saved in its new investigative zeal, but its focus on long stays and documentation has created offshoot hospice industries. Consultancies charge hospices big fees to train doctors, nurses, and pharmacists to fill out Medicare forms beyond reproach. Government contractors investigate hospices for inappropriate or poorly documented charges — and earn a percentage of the money recouped. This has turned Medicare audits into a form of bounty hunting. Government oversight is necessary, but the bureaucracy burdens every hospice. It recently destroyed San Diego Hospice, long considered one of the premier programs in the world.

The trouble started in 2011, when Medicare began an audit. As it dragged on for months and then years, hospice executives brought in a consultant to conduct an internal review. The findings could not have been worse. It was the consultant's opinion that the hospice kept patients in the program when they lived longer than expected — without the required documentation that their condition was getting worse. The consultant believed that without such documentation, the hospice would have no grounds to appeal allegations of overcharges or a government demand to pay back millions of dollars. It would be like getting caught by the I.R.S. without receipts for expenses you deducted.

The hospice's broad interpretation of its mission left it vulnerable. The program had always pushed the envelope on hospice care — it provided the full array of palliative treatments, including radiation, chemotherapy, and psychiatry. Contrary to the consultant's opinion, the medical staff insisted that they had followed the law, which requires doctors to periodically recertify patients who outlive the six-month prognosis. The medical staff contended that doctors had to explain why they believed a patient was still likely to die within six months, based on a physical exam and lab tests. But for recertification, doctors did not have to show that the patient was home-bound or continuing to deteriorate. Although auditors and consultants looked for such evidence to easily determine whether someone was terminal, by Medicare's definition, the medical staff said the law did not require it.

Maybe San Diego's administrative or financial lapses ran deeper. It was hard to know because, as of March 2013, Medicare still had not released its audit results. But it did not have to, because San Diego Hospice filed for bankruptcy and announced it was shutting down.

You can argue that rules are rules — that a hospice accepting taxpayer money is ethically and legally bound to check every box on every form and to adhere to the strictest interpretation of patient eligibility. Some people made exactly that case online when news of San Diego's troubles leaked out. But in the palliative care community, the reaction was grief. A palliative care specialist who blogs as Hospice Doctor, wrote: "At a time when there is universal consensus that we need more and better palliative care, the loss of this remarkable institution is, pure and simple, an unmitigated tragedy."

Scripps Health, a major nonprofit health care system in the region, bought San Diego Hospice's shuttered inpatient center and eight-acre hilltop campus, at a bankruptcy auction, for $16.55 million. Scripps CEO Chris Van Gorder publicly pledged a commitment "to sustaining the legacy" of the "visionaries" who founded and grew the hospice, going back to Doris Howell, a disciple of Cicely Saunders. Scripps planned to reopen the inpatient building in 2014.

The government's focus on long stays overlooks and in some ways feeds the biggest problem for patients: short hospice stays. Even as chains saturate communities with hospices — and even as nonprofits struggle to survive, with or without Hugh Westbrook's help — too many people do not receive the care they need because they come to hospice too late.

To its credit, the federal government is

taking tentative steps to change that. Under the Patient Protection and Affordable Care Act, better known as Obamacare, the government is funding demonstration projects around the country to test a concept called "concurrent care." This allows patients to enroll in hospice even if they want to continue potentially curative treatments. It eliminates the "cure versus care" dilemma that has shadowed hospice from the start.

Aetna, the giant health plan, liberalized its hospice benefit along these lines in 2004 for non-Medicare patients, with striking results. Aetna extended the definition of terminal illness from six months to twelve months. It lifted restrictions on how long patients can receive inpatient hospice care. Most significantly, the company did not compel patients to agree in writing to forego curative treatment as a condition of hospice admission — as Medicare has always done.

"We have pretty clearly demonstrated that this is an unnecessary barrier," said Randall Krakauer, Aetna's national Medicare medical director. "It serves no useful purpose and should be eliminated."

Aetna coupled its looser rules and expanded benefits with telephone support by nurses trained in palliative care. They provide "a lifeline" to vulnerable patients,

Krakauer said. Hospice use more than doubled, to 70 percent of eligible patients. And patients came to hospice care earlier, staying thirty-seven days on average, up from twenty-one days under the old rules. "It's still not long enough," Krakauer said, but the number has continued to inch up since the original study was completed.

Even though hospice patients had the option of pursuing curative or life-prolonging treatments, few seemed to do so. This is important because it suggests that allowing dying patients to keep this option eases their reluctance to enroll in hospice, but they do not flock to high-priced therapies once they receive comfort care. In other words, health costs will not skyrocket if Medicare stops forcing patients to give up life-prolonging treatments to receive hospice services. Medicare even may save money. Under Aetna's liberalized hospice benefit, patients made fewer trips to doctors and emergency rooms and spent less time in the hospital.

It will be years before the government collects the data on its concurrent care projects. Meanwhile, short hospice stays not only hurt patients and families; they also waste taxpayer money — more money, in fact, than long stays waste. In 2011, more than one-third of hospice patients died within a week of admission, which means that many received expensive aggressive treatment until the very end. In 2009, Medicare paid $55 billion in doctor and hospital bills during the final two months of patients' lives, more than four times what it paid for hospice care. An estimated 20 to 30 percent of those expenses produced no meaningful benefit.

Patients and families have every right to stick with aggressive treatment, fully informed about the side effects and its likely outcome. But many people, like Fred Holliday, come to hospice late because their doctors never tell them forthrightly that their illness is terminal. Or, like Rusty Hammer, they undergo agonizing treatments past the point of futility because their doctors oversell the potential benefits.

Or they do not come at all, because hospices themselves have never reached out.

Chapter Thirteen: Cultural Revolutions

"We don't just visit. We live there."

Hospice of Santa Cruz County, California, nestles in a redwood grove at the end of a cul-de-sac. While peaceful and lovely, the building is inaccessible to the large and growing population of Latino families who live in or near the city of Watsonville, twenty miles away. That's why the nonprofit hospice rented a building in Watsonville, next to the area's largest hospital, and opened the Center for End-of-Life Care in March 2013. The new offices serve as a base for Spanish-speaking hospice staff, and community members go there for educational events, trainings and grief support. Stacks of a photo-novella, *Una Historia de Hospice,* greet visitors.

An inability to attract communities of color has been the greatest failing of the hospice movement. In its neglect, hospice has not been that different from the health care system overall, and the failure reflects economic and social inequities etched into the American landscape. Still, the movement that was so far-sighted in embracing the social, emotional, and psychological aspects of health and well-being, so expansive in its services, has had a blind spot regarding race and ethnicity. People of color are the fastest growing populations in America, and by mid-century they will represent the majority. Yet more than 80 percent of hospice patients are white. They are much more likely to have heard about hospice through a relative or friend — somebody they trust who'd had a good experience with a program. People of color typically learn about hospice in the hospital, from a stranger. A 2007 study summed up a common reaction among Latinos: "I didn't know what hospice was. I thought it was a place worse than a hospital."

Hospice pioneers battled such misconceptions but most did not venture beyond their white middle-class worlds. Hospice of Santa Cruz founders began their meetings seated in a Buddhist prayer circle, chanting together for good health. In 1978, target marketing and diversifying the client base were not on the agenda, nor were they for most hospices until recently.

Now hospice websites may offer a half-dozen or more language options. Some sponsor events, such as Thanksgiving dinner, in underserved communities as a form of outreach. And many hospices employ cultural liaisons like Silvia Austerlic.

Austerlic was looking for a green card, not a career in hospice, when she took an internship at Hospice of Santa Cruz County. At thirty-two, she had come from Argentina, where unemployment topped 25 percent in the late 1990s. She had a student visa and taught Spanish to adults. But to stay in the country and for her own sense of purpose, she needed to be sponsored by an agency that could employ her skills to make a difference. While she was working on a master's degree in counseling education, Hospice of Santa Cruz County started to notice its lack of diversity and hired her to help find the reason for it.

The county's Latino population had grown to 33 percent, but only 3 percent of the hospice's patients were Latinos. Like Austerlic, most were immigrants looking to work for a better life. Many found work in the lettuce, strawberry, and artichoke fields that feed much of America. Also like Austerlic, most immigrants were young, which was one reason they never crossed paths with hospice.

But agricultural work is one of the most dangerous occupations in the United States. Farm workers suffer high rates of lung infections, serious respiratory ailments, and certain cancers, including brain and stomach cancers. To help the community participate in the benefits of hospice involves bridging the gap between lettuce fields and redwood grove. To Austerlic, it is not a matter of saying, "Oh, let us give you quality of life." It is: "Tell us what you need. Quality of life comes from within. We are really good at pain management, but we are also offering just to be there."

Having a visible presence in Watsonville carries that out, she said, "like bringing a casserole to a neighbor. We don't just visit. We live here."

A consistent barrier to hospice is that nobody likes to talk about death. We all have that in common. We avoid the conversation, whether in English, Cantonese, or Spanish, and getting there can be rocky. It was for the Ramirez family in Santa Cruz.

Maria de Lourdes Ramirez was diagnosed with breast cancer, and had a partial mastectomy and nine pretty good years. But in November 2005, despite the rounds of chemotherapy and radiation, her cancer had spread and was inoperable. Her children and grandchildren were shocked. Even when most of them could take it in, and Lourdes agreed to enroll in hospice so that she could remain at home, there was one adamant holdout.

Lourdes would say to her husband, Apolonio: *"Viejo, me voy a morir."* ("Old man" — but in a loving way, like "Honey" — "I am going to die.")

And he would say: *"No, no, no te vas a morir!"* ("No, no, you're not going to die!")

Later, Apolonio asked their eldest child, Irma Vega: Why did your mother never ask me to take care of the family when she was gone?

How could she, Irma thought, when he wouldn't even acknowledge that she was dying? Irma and her siblings meanwhile struggled with their own denial. As children they would say, "If Mamá dies. If Papá dies." When it was about to happen, Irma wasn't alone in thinking, "You mean it wasn't an *if*?"

Apolonio and Lourdes came from Guanajuato, Mexico, and their conversations and their children's assumptions would have sounded familiar to many Latino families. In a paper on medical ethics, Austerlic wrote, "Death and dying are topics that many Latinos may not be willing openly to discuss, especially when a loved one is seriously ill. As health deteriorates and there is a health crisis, families usually call 911 and/or rush to the emergency room or the hospital, wanting 'everything done.' "

The couple's conversations also would have sounded familiar to Sandy Chen Stokes, founder of the Chinese American Coalition for Compassionate Care. "Chinese culture demands that we do everything we can for a dying loved one," Chen Stokes said. "We want to be with our loved one as long as we can." Chinese Americans are five times more likely than Caucasians to die with feeding tubes. They are less likely to be removed from life support. They also are less likely to consent to pain medications such as morphine, because of the family's fear of addiction, deeply rooted in the nineteenth-century opium Wars, which devastated traditional culture in China and destroyed the nation's self-sufficiency for a century.

The Chinese tradition has been that families do not speak about death with the loved one who is dying unless she or he wants to, which they rarely do. "Talking is tantamount to cursing the person to death," said psychologist Wei-Chien Lee. Even today, adult children may ask doctors to soften bad news to the patient. If she or he does not speak English well, the family may avoid translating certain aspects of a grim medical situation.

In a DVD for the Chinese American Coalition for Compassionate Care, Lee recalled her father's final two years, suffering from a genetic disease. She wanted to tell him, "Thank you for working so hard in this life to care for us," and how sad she felt to see him so sick. She never got the chance. Ten years after he died, Lee found a note her dad wrote her: "My big regret in my entire life was that I never told you how much I love you."

For African Americans, barriers to health care in general — and to compassionate care in particular — are rooted in the harsh history of racism and economic inequality. African Americans have disproportionately high rates of infant mortality. African American women are less likely than white women to be diagnosed with cancer, but more likely to die from it. African American men have the highest risks of any group of developing most major cancers and dying from them. But hospice use by African Americans is low, about 11 percent.

African Americans often have a tradition of family decision-making that favors aggressive medical treatment, and disproportionately they die in ICUs. For them and for Latinos, religious beliefs about God's will and a distrust of doctors, rooted for some African Americans in the notorious Tuskegee Syphilis Study, also discourage hospice enrollment.

"It's Time to Call Hospice."
On a rainy day in November 2005, four members of the Ramirez family huddled with Jennifer Choate, Lourdes's oncologist. In contrast to much of their experience with medicine, this doctor spoke to them warmly and respectfully. Now she had to tell them Lourdes's cancer was back and, "I think it's time to call hospice."

Nobody knew what that meant. After a brief explanation, Irma, then age forty-eight, said, "Do we have to?"

They made medical decisions as a family and now second-guessed themselves. Had they been too eager to embrace whatever medical technology had to offer? Not aggressive enough? Maybe Mamá should have had the full mastectomy, as one surgeon recommended. Maybe she should have stopped chemo earlier. It made her so sick and in the end didn't work.

Choate reassured them that they did not have to do anything right then, that they had choices. They might want to try a support program called Transitions, sponsored by Hospice of Santa Cruz, for families facing serious illnesses. It would cover the basics, like understanding how the disease would progress, setting goals for the patient, making a plan and schedule for caregivers, and having advance health care directives on file.

Lourdes had been in the emergency department at Dominican Hospital repeatedly that fall. At five-foot-six, she weighed 200 pounds, had high blood pressure and diabetes, and had had several mini-strokes. A few days before Christmas, she had another mini-stroke and could not get up, her legs so painfully swollen that Irma worried her skin would tear. She went to the hospital again.

Once stabilized, Lourdes kept asking when she could go home. The whole family always came to their house on Christmas. Lourdes always made tamales and *champurrado,* a thick Mexican hot chocolate.

Sprung free on Christmas Eve, the large

Ramirez delegation at Dominican Hospital called the rest of the family to gather at Mamá's and Papá's. When the first few cars arrived at the house, Apolonio and Lourdes weren't there. Weak as she was, she had insisted on stopping at the grocery store for gallons of milk to make the *champurrado*.

Talking with the Transitions social worker had helped assure most of the family that, if Lourdes wanted to be home, hospice was the best option. Except for Apolonio. He could abide the general notion of the "do not resuscitate" form — that nobody would try to revive her if her heart stopped or she could no longer breathe. He went through the motions, agreeing to move into a spare bedroom so they could bring a twin bed in with Lourdes, so somebody could always be with her, but he refused to accept that she was dying.

For a time, the siblings too tried to protect their mother from the truth. Early on, after a volunteer from hospice left, Lourdes told her youngest son, Donnie, *"Mijo, ya estuvo."* ("Son, that's it.") She was letting him know she knew she was dying, but Donnie quickly said, oh no, that woman was just a visitor.

She snapped at him, *"No me mientas!"* ("Don't lie to me.")

A sheriff's deputy, Donnie knew all about

DNRs, but he had never imagined having to deal personally with their restrictions. At first he found himself hoping his mother would die on somebody else's watch. Then he thought, no, it would be better if he could be with her because, for the others, death could be shocking. Then again, maybe they would not fight it as hard as he would, to let her go. Trained as a first responder, Donnie had pumped on the chests and breathed into the mouths of strangers. Would he be able to stand by and let his own mother die?

His older brother Oscar, a policeman, struggled too. He had always been close to his mother, often calling her to ask, "Mamá, what should I do?" about matters big and small. Now he wondered how he could bathe his own mother, and change her bedding and diapers, as she had done for him so many years ago.

All in the Family

Apolonio Ramirez sent for his family in Guanajuato in 1961. He had a job at the Campbell's Soup mushroom farm in Pescadero, a farming community on the Central California coast between Santa Cruz and San Francisco. Lourdes found work that could be done at home, sorting and wiring dried flowers. It was slow, and paid only 30 cents a tray. But she did not speak English so could not get a teaching job, as she had in Mexico. To make more money, she went to work in the fields, and had to take her four preschool children with her.

Ten years later, they had saved enough to buy a three-bedroom house in Davenport, the house where she would die.

The siblings split up day and night shifts. They declined the help of an aide or chaplain, but Lourdes, a very private person, surprised everyone by welcoming a volunteer visitor from the hospice. Lourdes later told Irma she felt this woman was there just for her to confide in, without judgment.

Steeped in the tradition that only priests give Holy Communion, Lourdes had not been happy years earlier when Irma trained to become a Eucharist minister in their Catholic church, Our Lady Star of the Sea. Every Sunday morning, Irma served during the Mass at an assisted living facility and every Sunday, Lourdes asked, "Do you have to go?" About a month before she died, Lourdes asked, "Why do you give them the Holy Eucharist and not me?" Irma was thrilled to do it.

On her last day of life, March 25, 2006, Lourdes had a house full of visitors. It got a little loud, with grandchildren around and other relatives enjoying seeing each other and remembering old times. Irma went out and said the family needed to be alone.

Around ten o'clock that night, Lourdes's breathing got faster. They propped her up in bed, Donnie and Irma each holding a hand. Apolonio wanted to wait in the other room. Donnie struggled against his instinct to give her CPR. She jolted up with a very loud breath, then slowly her head fell back down, her hands went limp, and she was gone.

A hospice nurse came to remove the catheter, and left to let them spend the night alone before the rest of the family came to say farewell. Donnie made sure his mother was wearing her favorite Birkenstocks.

A few weeks later, Apolonio moved back into the bedroom, where he set up a little candle-lit shrine with photographs. He also signed a DNR. Still, he says that if he had known that enrolling in hospice meant death for sure, he never would have done it. Irma, meanwhile, became a hospice volunteer, trained to provide grief support for families like her own.

Hospices Reach Out

Silvia Austerlic, the Latino cultural liaison at Hospice of Santa Cruz, had spoken with Irma about "compassionate presence," just being with Lourdes in the days she had left. Being there for diverse communities requires more than translating the words of hospice into different languages. It requires a nuanced understanding of culture and values. Otherwise, hospice may look like withdrawing treatment and giving up hope.

Hospice of Santa Cruz has published *A Hospice Caring Story,* a photo-novella in Spanish and English, showing what hospice might look like for a woman who tells her friend, "I am so tired . . . taking care of my husband, the children, the house, and everything else. Besides, our family is in Mexico and I don't have anybody to help me!" Later, the hospice nurse tells the Moreno family, assembled on the couch, "We'll work with you and your doctor on a plan of care based on what you all need and what is important to your family."

Education must go two ways. Hospice staff need to know about *curanderismo,* folk healing practices, in case patients want to include its prayers, massages, and other rituals in their care. Doctors, nurses, and the rest of the team also need to understand cultural attitudes like the one that prompted a Latino study participant to say: "The worst thing about hospice care? The way they talk to you about death."

Austerlic understands. She said, "The whole idea of grieving is foreign. No, you suffer and move on. The Day of the Dead, yes, but not 'working through your grief.' " Traditions change, of course, with new generations and migration. First-generation Latino immigrants may get more solace from faith and rituals, while the third generation is more open to talking about feelings, and the second generation finds comfort in both.

Finally, a little language can be worse than none. The word *hospicio* looks like it means hospice, but historically it has referred to an orphanage, poorhouse, or place for the mentally ill. This is why the hospice's new office in Watsonville is called the Center for End-of-Life Care.

All this speaks to the urgent need for hospices to develop innovative, sensitive programs to serve their changing communities. Hospices will not survive unless they broaden their reach, and patients and families stand to benefit if they do.

The San Francisco Bay Area nonprofit Pathways Home Health & Hospice has fourteen languages represented on its staff, and brochures in English, Chinese, Spanish, Farsi, Tagalog, Russian, and Vietnamese. (And, helpfully for all, in large type.) A 2009 study of Pathways patients in Oakland found that a trial period of music therapy increased African American hospice enrollment from 15 percent to 25 percent. (African Americans account for 27 percent of the population of that city.) Music therapy not only attracted more patients, but also brought them tremendous comfort. By tapping into families' deep resonance with styles from gospel to jazz, the therapy reduced the use of medications and the need for nurses' visits. Families said it gave the patients something to look forward to, reduced their anxiety, and prompted memories. When the music therapy experiment ended, African American participation dropped to 17 percent.

In Broward County, Florida, Hospice by the Sea has long been considered one of the most innovative in the country. Founded by half a dozen volunteers in a Boca Raton storefront in 1978, the nonprofit now serves 4,000 patients a year. Among its 600 employees are African American community outreach coordinators in Broward and Palm Beach counties, who bring presentations about palliative and hospice care to local churches, clubs, and homeowners' associations.

A more recent arrival on the hospice scene is the nonprofit Pallium India USA. Founded in September 2010, it trains volunteers for hospice and works with organizations such as the Indo American Cancer Association, to provide culturally sensitive end-of-life information and care.

The point of programs like these is to build trust, a two-way street. As opposed to missionaries coming in to convert, or anthropologists to study, hospice's goal is to be a partner in care: not a stranger, not an outsider, but a neighbor.

CHAPTER FOURTEEN: NOT IF, BUT WHEN

"How you want to die is an interesting question as long as you're not about to die."

The hospice system is far from perfect, but the hospice philosophy has changed our country for the better. It has given us permission to talk about dying and a language to advocate for the care we want for ourselves and those we love. Hospice has shown that it is never too late to answer the question: What do you want to do with the rest of your life?

And it is never too early.

That's where the Go Wish card game, created by hospice physician Elizabeth Menkin, comes in. It is part of a growing effort to rethink how we plan for dying, just as hospice redefined how we care for it.

The packaging promises to give you "an easy, entertaining way to think and talk about what's important to you if you become seriously ill." The cards are designed like a kids' deck, in cheerful blocks of red, teal, and purple. Menkin produced them in conjunction with Coda Alliance, a California-based nonprofit organization working to improve end-of-life planning (and, as we saw in Chapter 6, she beta tested it on her father, Peter Serrell). A pack has thirty-six cards, each with a wish: To be pain-free or anxiety-free or free of the hospital. To have friends or family near. To have financial affairs in order. To be at peace with God. To maintain a sense of humor. You consider the possibilities until you have picked your top ten. It's available through Coda (www.codaalliance.org), in Spanish and English, $24 for two packs.

Tools like Go Wish steer planning for end-of-life care beyond the documents that we sign without much thought, if we sign them at all. Although forms like advance directives are important legally, they often do not help people make life-and-death health care decisions when the time comes. That's in large part because the documents say nothing about the kind of life or death you hope to have but focus instead on the medical instruments to be used or avoided. Do you want a feeding tube if you're terminally ill? CPR or a breathing machine? "It's like asking, do you want your car mechanic to use a torque wrench?" Menkin said. "You don't really care. You just want him to fix your car."

Go Wish helps people to identify what they value most in the end, so that those desires can guide the complicated health care choices that we all will face — or that our families will make for us. If your greatest wish is to live as long as possible, no matter what, a feeding tube or ventilator may make sense in certain circumstances. On the other hand, if you feel that life is worth living only as long as you can savor your food or have the strength and mobility to cradle your grandchild, you may decide at some point that you would be much better off on hospice.

Menkin's cards are just one way to get your brain around the possibilities. Many states have versions of POLST (physician orders for life-sustaining treatment), forms that specify instructions to hospitals and doctors. The Conversation Project (http://theconversationproject.org/), founded in 2012, encourages what the name says — lots of talk. The creator, former journalist Ellen Goodman, used to write a column syndicated in more than 300 newspapers.

Hers was a household name, and she is determined to make end-of-life wishes a kitchen-table conversation topic. A "starter kit" guides you, with questions to help you figure out just what kind of care you would want, and with icebreakers to help you bring up the subject with others. ("I need to think about the future. Will you help me?")

A Boston-based nonprofit organization, Engage With Grace, has distilled the choices ahead to one free slide that can be downloaded, emailed, or shared on Facebook (http://www.engagewithgrace.org/Questions .aspx). It asks five questions:

1. On a scale of 1 to 5, rank where you fall on this continuum: *Let me die without medical intervention* (1) to *Try any proven or unproven intervention possible* (5).

2. If there were a choice, would you prefer to die at home or in a hospital?

3. Could a loved one correctly describe how you'd want to be treated if you were terminally ill?

4. Is there someone you trust whom you've appointed to advocate on your behalf when the time is near?

5. Have you completed an advance care directive and other documents indicating what kind of care you want and who may make decisions for you?

Alexandra Drane, a health care communications executive, started Engage With Grace after the death of her thirty-two-year-old sister-in-law. Rosaria Vandenberg — everyone called her Za — had stage 4 glioblastoma, an aggressive brain cancer. She underwent two operations, radiation, and chemotherapy, and spent the last two months of her life in the hospital. Her husband finally took her home, with hospice help, over the objections of her medical team. The night she settled in, her two-year-old daughter crawled into bed beside her for the first time since Za had been hospitalized. Za died the next day.

It had been seven months from her diagnosis to her death. The average survival time for stage 4 glioblastoma without treatment is about five months. "We tortured my sister-in-law," Alexandra Drane said recently. "We didn't get her into hospice until very late. And I'm in the health care space, and I'm not a wimp. But I was so scared. We should have known that what she wanted to do was be with her daughter, but we had never talked about any of this, and we didn't advocate for her. We took what the system gave us."

Drane has presented her slide at TEDMED, the annual conference on emergent ideas in health care and technology. Every Thanksgiving, Engage With Grace holds a "blog rally," blasting the slide all over the Web to get families to pause between turkey and football to talk about what it means to them to die well. "People need to see this as something that's their right, their obligation, what it means to be part of humanity. They need to see there didn't used to be cool, sexy, social media people who thought that fixing end-of-life care mattered, and now there are," she said.

"How you want to die is an interesting question as long as you're not about to die."

Making Good Choices When the Time Comes

For every story like Drane's about doctors who hold on beyond reason, there is at least one tale of the family who refuses to let go no matter what the medical team advises. Doctors get stuck in the default mode, which is to treat. Insert the feeding tube. Hook up the breathing machine. Shock the heart back to action when it stops.

"There's such a difference between the family who has been talking about these things for twenty years and the people who are like deer caught in the headlights," said Rebecca Sudore, associate professor of medicine at the University of California, San Francisco, and a hospice and palliative care physician at the city's VA Medical Center. "You call a friend of a patient — the person who's named on the form as durable power of attorney, the person appointed to make decisions — and he says, 'What? Me? I haven't talked to that guy in five years.'"

Since her days as a medical student, Sudore has thought about "the disconnect" between the needs of the health care system and those of patients when it comes to making tough decisions about care. The bureaucracy needs standardized documents with quick indicators of the patient's treatment preferences — attorney-vetted forms to slip into the medical record, guide doctors, and protect them from getting sued. Patients and families need clear information about the illness and the likely benefits and physical and emotional tolls of treatment. "A checkbox is a checkbox is a checkbox," Sudore said. "It's not real life."

The standard paperwork — the advance directive, indicating what medical interventions you want, and the health care proxy or durable power of attorney, naming someone to make decisions on your behalf — generally gets signed once, if ever, and filed away. The documents remain fixed while life changes. Your proxy may be the spouse you divorced, acrimoniously, a decade ago. Or life-prolonging treatment may not seem as bad as it did in the abstract, now that the very real alternative is death.

Research shows that many people cannot imagine coping with a serious illness or disability and say they would want to forego aggressive therapies, but, when it happens, they are more willing to try invasive treatments, even with limited benefits. That shifts again as people age. Aggressive treatment for stage 3 breast cancer looks different to a woman at forty-six who has two teen-agers at home than to a ninety-two-year-old great-great grandmother who has lived a full life.

The language of advance directives can muddle decisions, and the jargon and legalese are only part of the problem. Directives often talk about foregoing interventions when a condition is "irreversible" or "terminal," a difficult and sometimes impossible determination for a doctor to make. The directive typically asks people to make serious medical decisions based on hypothetical future scenarios. When the real crisis occurs, it poses dilemmas that nobody anticipated.

To help patients understand the forms, Sudore created an advance directive at a fifth-grade reading level for California. (You can download it at www.iha4health.org.) But she soon realized that the forms were not enough — people also needed to be able to make the best decisions possible at the worst times of their lives. Then, at one of the worst times in her life, she had a conversation with her grandparents that shook her and changed her thinking about end-of-life planning. She wrote about the incident in an essay in the *Journal of the American Medical Association,* called "Can We Agree to Disagree?"

Her grandfather had diabetes, congestive heart failure, kidney trouble, and other serious medical problems when he fell, broke his hip, and underwent surgery. Over the next six months, he went back and forth between his nursing home and the hospital for treatment of a list of problems. As his condition got worse, Sudore asked his doctors to talk with both her grandparents about whether to continue this way. Nobody initiated that discussion, so she finally did.

"My grandfather was really clear," she recalled recently. "He said, 'I am tired and I am done. I've had a good life.' " He said he did not fear dying, and he did not want to be resuscitated or end up on life support.

As his designated decision-maker, Sudore's grandmother was equally clear about her desires. If he could no longer communicate his wishes, she would tell the doctors to do everything possible to keep him alive.

In the essay, Sudore described her consternation. Why would her grandmother ask for treatments that her husband did not want? "She told me that she loved my grandfather too much to let him go," Sudore wrote.

And how did he feel about the choices that his wife might make for him? Just fine, he assured Sudore — and this too shocked her. He explained that, above all, he hoped his wife would do whatever she needed, because she would have to live with her decision, Sudore wrote.

Eight years after the conversation, Sudore still choked up to recount it. At the time, it opened her eyes to a dynamic that traditional advance care planning had missed. The needs of the relative or friend appointed to make decisions may bear on the choices they will make, in ways that doctors and patients do not recognize. Even the best planning cannot take into account every possibility. Would you permit your decision-maker to override your written treatment preference, if that might make you more comfortable? Whose wishes should rule if your decision-maker desperately wants doctors to be more aggressive than you had previously stated — or, for that matter, less aggressive?

In early 2013, Sudore released a user-friendly interactive Web-based tool called PREPARE (www.prepareforyourcare.org). It walks you through a five-step process. Like Drane's slide, the site helps you to identify what's important to you if you're sick, and to appoint the right person to make decisions for you if you can't. It also helps you to decide how much flexibility to give that person in making those decisions, and it shows you how to ask doctors good questions. The tool prompts you to commit to an action plan, with a deadline, before logging off.

Of course, no tool works unless people use it. Only one-third to one-half of American adults have signed advance directives. (Doctors do better, but at 64 percent in one study even they fall short.) We overestimate the success of rescue efforts and underestimate the pain they can cause. The pioneers of modern CPR envisioned it as a technique to restore a "heart too good to die," not to restart a "heart too sick to live." Only 8 percent of people who suffer cardiac arrest outside the hospital are saved by CPR, and even in the hospital, only about one patient in five is revived. TV medical dramas love a good resuscitation scene, but we never see the paddles come out for a frail, very sick, very old patient or never hear the crunch of ribs cracking as doctors go to work.

A Harvard physician, Angelo Volandes, is beginning to prove that we would make different choices if we understood what life-prolonging treatments entail. He has created a series of short videos to show people what it's like to undergo CPR or have a breathing tube pushed down the throat. The videos are graphic, though sanitized — life-size dummies serve as the patients, leaving the mess, fright, and noise of the real experience to the viewer's imagination. Nevertheless, his research shows that the videos open people's eyes and change their minds. In a study of patients with advanced cancer, only 20 percent who viewed the CPR video said they would want the procedure if their heart stopped. Among patients who did not see the video, 48 percent said they would favor CPR.

Given how readily a public conversation

about these issues can degenerate into shouting about death panels, it's easy to imagine that widespread use of such videos would get some people screaming about a Harvard doc who wants to pull the plug on Granny. This misses a fundamental point: Signing an advance directive does not necessarily mean rejecting treatment. People can, and do, indicate on the forms that they want to be kept alive by all means possible. And, even if a person signs a "do not resuscitate" form, that does not rule out other treatments that may improve comfort and quality of life, such as pain medication, antibiotics, or even surgery. In any case, we are a long way from broad use of these videos. As of late 2012, only thirty-five of the nearly 6,000 hospitals in this country had ordered them.

Videos and horror stories are not the only way to motivate people to think about, or rethink, the care they hope to have. Research shows that witnessing a loved one die in peace, without pain, gives survivors a powerful impetus to tell their doctors and their families that they want that too. Lisa Renstrom, an environmentalist and nonprofit executive, thought about this in the weeks after her mother died of leukemia at home, with hospice care. It occurred to Renstrom that dying naturally isn't so different from giving birth that way, yet we prepare almost maniacally for the arrival of life while pretending the departure will never occur.

"In today's society you don't just *do* natural childbirth," she said. "You take classes, you read books, you tour the hospital, you practice the right way to breathe." And it's not only the mom who prepares. It's also her spouse, her birth coach, her sorority sisters — whoever will stand by her side. The prospect of a death, of course, does not hold the same joy and excitement, but the process demands no less focus and presence, and usually more. "It takes preparation," Renstrom said. "You don't just *be* with someone in their final days. It takes an investment of thought."

Like so many people, Lisa Renstrom learned this only after finding herself in the situation she had never anticipated, quitting her job to care for her seventy-seven-year-old mother at the family home in Charlotte, North Carolina. Lisa's daughter, Alex Mangimelli, and a family friend, Ada Garibay, moved in to help. They had terrifying moments that, in hindsight, they would have handled better if they'd known what was coming. A frightening episode of projectile vomiting prompted a panicked call to 911 and a hospital stay that nobody wanted. Lisa brought her mother home again, hired more help, and had long talks with the hospice nurse about how to deal with a crisis. Then the household settled into a tranquil routine.

Time seemed suspended. The women kept the bedroom bathed in candlelight and took turns by the bedside. Some nights, inside the bed, Lisa, then Alex, then Ada would squeeze around the two miniature poodles holding vigil on the mattress to lie beside and hug a woman they all dearly loved. Each day she seemed to shrink by half. Lisa was not religious, but like the Catholic Sisters who opened the nineteenth-century hospices in Dublin and London, she felt as if she was ushering her mother "through the door."

One morning, Ada shouted from the bedroom for Lisa and Alex to come. They watched Lisa's mother take her final breath, and then they stood frozen, not sure what to do next. At last, someone turned on music.

Michael Bublé's jazzy, exuberant version of the song "Feeling Good" filled the house. To brassy orchestration, Bublé sang of a new dawn, a new day, a new life. They played it again and again, maybe twelve times. "We decided that she had chosen it for us and for herself," Lisa would say later. Lisa called the hospice, and a nurse arrived quickly. She told the women to go for a walk while she waited for the funeral director to pick up the body. Lisa watched as the nurse dressed her mother in her favorite beige and black plaid Burberry blouse, and then the three women left the house.

They wandered around, not saying much. As they headed home, the nurse drove up, waved, rolled down the window, and cranked up Michael Bublé on the car stereo. Lisa smiled.

REFLECTIONS

We started this book intent on answering a question we kept hearing from people who had experienced hospice: Why can't the rest of health care be like this? Through doctors and families we met and stories we heard, we found many reasons to hope that hospice principles are bringing health care closer to the model of compassionate care. We also came away hopeful that dying with dignity, whatever that means to any one of us, can become the national standard.

Then there were the surprises for each of us.

FRAN: As we were racing to finish the proposal for this book and send it to our agent, I was diagnosed with breast cancer.

It was caught early, stage 0, ductal carcinoma in situ. Some experts — notably, Susan Love, the well-known breast cancer specialist and patient advocate — do not even call it cancer but pre-cancer, because the abnormal cells are just sitting there. They haven't invaded the surrounding tissue, cancer's hallmark, and they may never. But because they might, the standard protocol is to treat it like a more advanced cancer, in my case with surgery and radiation.

I'm sure my doctor told me all this when she called me on my cell phone to break the news. But my shock seemed to scramble my capacity to make sense of her words. I was in the passenger seat of a rental car rounding a freeway ramp out of San Francisco International Airport, and my upper body began to shake. Behind the wheel, my husband performed the amazing feat of keeping his eyes on the road while never taking them off me. The doctor said something about the cure rate or success rate being 99 percent. She told me not to worry or rush home to New York, just enjoy the trip and call her when I returned.

I had lots of crazy thoughts that night, including this: Did taking on a book about hospice, venturing into the world of death and dying, somehow bring on my diagnosis?

Two days later, Sheila and I sat in the sunny, immaculate living room of Jerry Farnsworth and Shirley Gregory, who had met in a bereavement group and later married. Jerry mentioned that his first wife had died of breast cancer, and my stomach seized. She had been treated for it successfully twenty years earlier. "Everybody forgot" she'd ever had it, he said with a sad shake of his head. Needless to say, they remembered when it recurred and killed her. I jotted notes, nodding empathetically while, inside, crazies screamed: Leave now. Stop talking about this stuff. You're asking for trouble.

Of course, the random universe does not work that way. Thinking about death and spending time with dying patients will not make you die. That's going to happen, no matter what. I'm not saying anything I didn't know going into this project. But I really got it, somewhere deep, spending time with very sick people. The only difference between them and me, between their families and mine, was a terminal diagnosis. I'm paraphrasing Susan Love, who made the point in a speech to scientists not long ago. She was trying to nudge them out of their zone of detachment to pay more attention to the human needs of people with cancer. "The only difference between a researcher and a patient is a diagnosis," the *New York Times* quoted her as saying. "We're all

341

patients." Just a few months later, Love was diagnosed with leukemia.

As Sheila and I wrote in the introduction, our fathers' deaths and our conversations about our different experiences planted the seeds for this book. My father spent nearly ten years slipping away, and I later wondered whether hospice would have made it better, faster, easier. I see now that behind that question was magical thinking and an all-too-common misconception about how hospice works. I envisioned hospice people swooping in, cleaning up his messes, grinding up his pills, soothing him back to sleep when he woke up shouting at four o'clock in the morning. Basically, I imagined them lifting the physical and emotional load that weighed so heavily on my mother.

Instead I discovered that hospice is pretty much do-it-yourself care. Countless families bear the same burdens my mother did, even with hospice support. We often refer to aggressive high-tech treatments as "heroic" measures, but the real heroics take place in the living room of a ranch house or the bedroom of a small apartment, when a family tends to the care and comfort of a dying loved one. This is not to say that hospice doesn't do much — it is a gift. But what it does best is help people face the unfathomable with grace, courage, and love, and to let them know that, at the saddest, scariest, most isolating time of their lives, they are not alone. I talked with many people who mourned the loss of a parent, sibling, spouse, or dear friend, but felt grateful for and transformed by the experience of helping that person pass.

I am not religious, but I came to think of hospice as sacred work. Spending time in a house where someone is dying — watching a doctor or nurse inspect his skin for sores or swelling, listen to her heartbeat, attend to the needs of a grieving family — always reminded me to take in life fully. To pay attention to the practical and the mysterious, to the universal and the personal, to what can be said in words and what remains in the heart.

SHEILA: "When you die, can I have your red shoes?" Shoes were the focus of my daughter's interest in mortality at age five.

Two decades later, she is more realistic. Now, she pleads, "Can we please talk about something else?" During the two years Fran and I spent researching and writing about hospice, Lisa often walked into a house filled with books like *Dying Well* and *Final Gifts,* phone interviews about congestive

343

heart failure and oxygen concentrators, and my husband and I talking about whether it was more important to die at home or to not be gasping for breath. When we played Go Wish cards to rank our end-of-life desires, Lisa wailed, "I don't like this game!"

As we all came to see, Ned and I weren't going to die earlier just because we talked about it. Hospice sources often mentioned the importance of having your advance health care directives in order, which loomed as an impossibly complicated and painful project until Ned reminded me that we already had done it. More than a decade ago, the attorney who drew up our trust papers had insisted.

Besides discovering that we'd already accomplished something very important for our children, and that our end-of-life choices hadn't changed, I have been surprised by what happens when you focus on the question, "What do you want to do with the rest of your life?"

Often, I clutch. What a question. As when my children were babies and they'd fall asleep, I'd run through a list of what to do before they woke up: Quick, take a nap. Wait, wash the dishes. No, read a book about childcare! Now, again, what is most important to do before time runs out?

I heard Maurice Sendak talking to Terry Gross on National Public Radio in a wonderful interview in 2011: "I have nothing now but praise for my life. I'm not unhappy. I cry a lot because I miss people. . . . They die and I can't stop them. They leave me and I love them more. . . . Oh God, there are so many beautiful things in the world which I will have to leave when I die, but I'm ready, I'm ready, I'm ready."

I'm not ready. Every year, naturally, we go to more funerals. Every year, as author Stephen Kiernan says in the DVD *Consider the Conversation*, I pass what will be the anniversary of my death.

I like to think I'm more understanding of my mother; she is eighty-four and in good shape, and this year we took a great trip to Cuba together. But looking on the bright side has never been her nature, my father's long decline didn't help, and, well, she's my mother. She lives in a large retirement community where illness and death are not shocking occurrences. Her news of the day often begins with a shout-out to Bette Davis: "Old age is no place for sissies." I used to tune out, or get annoyed and snap, "How many times do you have to say that?" And then I'd call my sister to complain about Mom.

At first out of professional interest for this book, I listened. Everyone she knows is falling off the treadmill; this is what it's like to wait your turn. She is afraid, naturally, and very willing to talk about what she wants and doesn't want, as she sees ever more instances of each. I'm grateful that she has all the advance directives in order, but I'm worried about what is actually going to happen.

From the beloved group of bereaved spouses profiled in this book, I saw how life can go on, even joyfully. And that losing a parent does not prepare you for losing a spouse, any more than raising a dog prepares you to raise children.

I learned that it doesn't have to be depressing for old people to die. They are like movies and novels, with great stories about what they've done in their lives. Hospice doctor Ellen Brown sees this all the time with the medical students she takes on home visits. "At first glance they might say, 'I wouldn't want to live like that. Old, decrepit, knowing I'm going to die.' But then they see that people do."

Everybody has a different idea of what they want and a different way of facing it, like Moses and Aaron in the Bible. Brown had two patients who lived the contrast.

One was a tragedy, a woman in her late fifties with ALS, confined to a wheelchair and feeding tube. "She couldn't do anything," Brown said. "But she enjoyed watching her grandchildren play." The other patient was twenty years older but in better shape. "She didn't want friends to see her because she was drooling. She was ready to die."

Finally, my sense of spirituality is evolving. I learned that it's OK to hedge your bets. Who knows? As Maurice Sendak said when asked if he was still stridently irreligious now that he was close to death: "I don't believe in an afterlife. But I fully expect to see my brother again."

And he laughed.

ACKNOWLEDGMENTS

Our foremost gratitude goes to the many families who welcomed us into their lives at a very difficult time. We are also grateful to those who revisited a time of loss to share their stories and their perspectives on hospice. Only a few of the dozens of families we interviewed appear in this book, but every one helped us immensely. Again and again, they showed us that no two families, and often no two people within a family, experience hospice the same way.

Karen Storey, our friend and former colleague at the *San Jose Mercury News,* led us to the Hospice of the Valley bereavement group, whose members opened many other doors. Elizabeth Menkin was unfailingly generous with her time, wisdom, and contacts, and she fed us well whenever we came to town. Ellen Brown took us on home visits and answered endless questions. Our thanks to the professionals and advocates who guided us through the hospice world, past and present — Sally Adelus, Tom Alain, Cathy Conway, Dale Larson, Shelly Marder, Mike Milward, Jeanne Wun, Edmund Sacks, Hugh Westbrook, Mychal Springer, Regina Holliday, Alexandra Drane, Rebecca Sudore, Cynthia Adams, Deborah Carr, Jamie Floyd, Roy Remer, Patty Riley, Ilene Scharlach, Andy Scharlach, Chris Taich, Mary Taverna, and Madalon Amenta.

The Hospice and Palliative Care Oral History, a global archive at the School of Interdisciplinary Studies at the University of Glasgow, Dumfries Campus, was a treasure trove of information on Cicely Saunders, Florence Wald, and other hospice pioneers. Very special thanks to David Clark for making transcripts available to us before the archive was fully open. Sister Mary de Paul welcomed us to the archives of the Dominican Sisters of Hawthorne, which houses the papers of Rose Hawthorne Lathrop and Alice Huber. The Florence and Henry Wald Papers and the Edward F. Dobihal Jr. Papers at Yale University shed light on the struggles to establish the first hospice in America. This book would not have been possible without the rich repository of material at the New York Public Library and its free online access to dozens of medical journals.

We are indebted to Karin Klein for invaluable advice on the manuscript. Patricia Albers, Susan Cohen, Amy Furth, Paulette Kessler, Linda Gray Sexton, Larry Slonaker, and Milly Hawk Daniel read chapter drafts and made wise suggestions. Pete Carey and Lisa Krieger provided helpful guidance on reporting. Connie Casey and Harold Varmus gave us the gift of paradise — a week to work without distraction at their beautiful cottage.

Thank you to John Rudolph of Dystel & Goderich Literary Management, who helped us shape an idea into the makings of a book. Thank you to Brenda Knight, our sharp, passionate editor and publisher at Viva Editions. Thanks also to Kara Wuest and the rest of the expert, enthusiastic team at Viva. Thanks to Kitty Burns Florey for her copyediting.

We spent more than two years in the hospice world, and every day reminded us that nothing matters more than the people in our lives. Our families supported us in more ways than we can say. FRAN: My mother, Dorothy Smith, showed me what it means to care for a loved one through death. My husband, David Yarnold, championed this project at every step, read endless drafts, and never came home from a business trip — or a golf trip — without some new hospice contact for me. Our daughter, Nicole, cheered me on, filling our home with music and laughter. SHEILA: My mother, Elaine Highiet, taught me the value of community. My husband, Ned Himmel, tapped his expert research skills to find archives, journals, and documents we needed — and kept me well nourished in all the important ways. Our children, Jake and Lisa, give me the reason to write.

All the names, places, and events in this book are real. Any errors are our own.

NOTES

Introduction
44 percent of all deaths. A $14 billion industry National Hospice and Palliative Care Organization, *NHPCO Facts and Figures: Hospice Care in America,* accessed March 13, 2013, http://www.nhpco.org/sites/default/files/public/Statistics_Research/2012_Facts_Figures.pdf.

Chapter 1: What Do You Want to Do with the Rest of Your Life?
March 2011 poll of 1,000 adults "New Poll: Americans Choose Quality over Quantity at the End of Life, Crave Deeper Public Discussion of Health Care Options," PRNewswire, last modified March 8, 2011, http://www.prnewswire.com/news-releases/new-poll-americans-choose-quality-over-quantity-at-the-end-of-life-crave-deeper-public-discussion-of-care-options-117575453.html.

fifty-nine hospice programs served patients and **1981 directory of the fledgling National Hospice Organization** David S. Greer, Vincent Mor et al., "National Hospice Study Analysis Plan," *Journal of Chronic Diseases,* 36, no. 11 (1983): 737-780.

hospice use among Medicare patients nearly doubled Joan M. Teno, Pedro L. Gozalo, Julie P.W. Bynum et al., "Change in End-of-Life Care for Medicare Beneficiaries, Site of Death, Place of Care, Health Care Transitions in 2000, 2005, and 2009," *Journal of the American Medical Association,* 309, no. 5 (2013): 470–477.

median length of service is just nineteen days. Thirty-six percent of hospice patients die within a week National Hospice and Palliative Care Organization, *NHPCO Facts and Figures.*

At the age of eighteen, he had been voted onto the city council "Teen Elected to Campbell Council," *San Jose Mercury,* April 12, 1972.

In 1975, he became the nation's youngest mayor ever elected Jose Stell, "Hammer Gets Gavel at 21," *San Jose Mercury,* March 13, 1975.

For once, the tabloid downplayed the story Dan McDonald, "Youngest Mayor Is

Only 22," *National Enquirer,* March 1975.

All I wanted to do was go home for good Rusty Hammer, *When Cancer Calls . . . Say Yes to Life: The Story of One Man's Journey through Leukemia* (Bloomington, Indiana: iUniverse, 2007).

bring a baby elephant to visit Shirley du Boulay. Updated by Marianne Rankin. *Cicely Saunders: The Founder of the Modern Hospice Movement* (London: SPCK Publishing, 2007).

the antimatter of cancer therapy Siddhartha Mukherjee, *The Emperor of All Maladies: A Biography of Cancer* (New York: Scribner, 2010).

We were most naïve about the side effects and risks of treatment at the various stages Hammer, *When Cancer Calls . . . Say Yes to Life.*

Chapter 2: Birth of a Movement
I've got the wrong slide Doris Howell interview, October 25, 1997, Hospice and Palliative Care Oral History Archive, School of Interdisciplinary Studies, University of Glasgow, Dumfries Campus.

Constant pain needed constant control Sister Mary Antonia interview, November 28, 1995, Hospice and Palliative Care Oral History Archive, School of Interdisciplinary Studies, University of Glasgow, Dumfries Campus.

Put this toward more wine Cicely Saunders to Christopher Saunders, July 6, 1965, in *Cicely Saunders: Founder of the Hospice Movement: Selected Letters 1959–1999,* ed. David Clark (Oxford: Oxford University Press, 2002).

never-ending intensive treatment carried to the bitter end Florence Wald, "The Emergence of Hospice Care in the United States," in *Facing Death: Where Culture, Religion, and Medicine Meet,* ed. Howard M. Spiro, Mary G. McCrea Curnen, Lee Palmer Wandel (New Haven: Yale University Press, 1998).

Our Lady's Hospice in Dublin in 1879 Clare Humphreys, " 'Waiting for the Last Summons': The Establishment of the First Hospices in England 1878–1914," *Mortality* 6, no. 2 (2001): 146–166. Also, Joy Buck, "Reweaving a Tapestry of Care: Religion, Nursing, and the Meaning of Hospice, 1945–1978," *Nursing History Review* 15 (2007): 113–145. Also, Cicely Saunders interview, May 11, 2004, Centenary History St. Joseph's Hospice, Hospice and Palliative Care Oral History Archive, School of Interdisciplinary Studies, University of Glasgow, Dumfries Campus.

Death was an obsession James Stevens Curl, *The Victorian Celebration of Death* (London: The History Press, 2001). Also, Philippe Ariès, *The Hour of Our Death: The Classic History of Western Attitudes Toward Death over the Last One Thousand Years,* trans. Helen Weaver (New York: Sterling Publishing, 2000).

The care the English take of all particulars Amoret Tanner, *"Funeralia in Excelsis,"* the Ephemera Society, last modified 2003, http://www.ephemerasociety.org.uk/articles/funeralia.html.

They died in conditions worse than the most savage M. D. Stenson, "Waiting for the Last Summons: A Work of God's Love," *The Catholic Fireside,* 1913, pp. 344–45, quoted in Humphreys, "Waiting for the Last Summons."

as comfortable and happy as if their own people Report of the Homes of the Servants of Relief for Incurable Cancer, Sisters of the Dominican Order, 1913, *The Rose Hawthorne Guild* 4, no. 1 (Summer 2009): accessed March 20, 2013, http://www.hawthorne-dominicans.org/guild/Guild%20News%20Letter%20V4%20N1.pdf.

the best treatment of all Ibid.

The men will ask to venture outdoors Ibid.

It is a mistake to erect a hospital Sister Mary Alphonsa Lathrop, "Sacrifices for the Poor — A Difficulty Challenged," *Christ's Poor* 1 no.10, May 1902, quoted in Diana Culbertson, ed., *Rose Hawthorne Lathrop Selected Writings* (Mahwah, NJ: Paulist Press, 1993).

Incurable cancer is now a matter of general and exhaustive study Ibid.

innate patrician and **Ugliness, dirt, disharmony revolted her** Julian Hawthorne, "A Daughter of Hawthorne," *Atlantic Monthly,* 142, no. 000003 (September 1928): 372–377.

Nothing less than the extreme would satisfy Ibid.

As best I can, I am answering the question Maurice Francis Egan, "A Legacy from Hawthorne," *New York Times Book Review and Magazine,* Apr. 16, 1922.

half a face relinquished to the disease Sister Mary Alphonsa Lathrop, "First Case Received by the Charity for Cancerous Poor." *Christ's Poor* 1, no. 2, September 1901.

Kind friend, the baby is dead Mrs. McNamara to Rose Hawthorne Lathrop,

Aug. 11, 1897. Rose Hawthorne Lathrop Papers, Dominican Sisters of Hawthorne Archive, Hawthorne, NY.

I loathed everything about the place M. Rose Huber, "A Brief History of the Work," 1936, Mother M. Rose Huber Papers, Dominican Sisters of Hawthorne Archive, Hawthorne, NY.

I asked what I had to do to say thank you and serve Saunders, *Cicely Saunders.* Also, David Clark, "Religion, Medicine, and Community in the Early Origins of St. Christopher's Hospice," *Journal of Palliative Medicine* 4, no. 3 (July 7, 2004).

David Tasma told me of the difficulties Cicely Saunders, "Hospice — A Meeting Place for Religion and Science," in *Cicely Saunders: Selected Writings 1958–2004* (Oxford: Oxford University Press, 2006).

I only want what is in your mind and your heart Cicely Saunders, "A Place to Die," *Crux* 11, no. 3 (1973–4): 24–27, in Saunders, *Cicely Saunders.*

It is the doctors who desert the dying Cicely Saunders, "Origins: International Perspectives — Then and Now," *Hospice Journal* 14, no. 3/4 (1999): 1–7.

I began to realize, as I listened to patients Saunders, "Hospice," in *Cicely*

Saunders.

virtually untouched by medical advance and support Ibid. Also, Cicely Saunders interviews, October 24, 1995–July 10, 1996, Hospice and Palliative Care Oral History Archive, School of Interdisciplinary Studies, University of Glasgow, Dumfries Campus. Also, Cicely Saunders, "Working at St. Joseph's Hospice, Hackney," Annual Report of St. Vincent's, Dublin, in Saunders, *Cicely Saunders,* 37–39.

it was like manna from heaven Sister Mary Antonia interview, November 28, 1995, Hospice and Palliative Care Oral History Archive, School of Interdisciplinary Studies, University of Glasgow, Dumfries Campus.

My father's complaint was that the Church Florence Wald interview by Monica Mills, June 10, 2003, Oral History Archive, Connecticut Women's Hall of Fame, accessed March 30, 2013, http://www.cwhf .org/media/upload/files/Transcripts/Wald% 20Interview%20Transcript.pdf.

collaboratively rather than competitively or antithetically Florence Wald, "Alternatives in the Care for the Terminally Ill," November 8, 1978, paper prepared for the U.S. Department of Health, Education and Welfare, Florence and Henry Wald Papers, Yale University, New Haven, Connecticut.

once stunned a room full of medical students at the University of Colorado Christopher Phillips, "To Be Whole Again," *Parade Magazine,* August 11, 1991, 11–12.

may cry for rest, peace, and dignity Elisabeth Kübler-Ross, *On Death and Dying* (New York: Scribner, 1997).

established an account at Orange National Bank with a $142.50 deposit Lawrence L. Kerns, "A Study of the Creation of a Community Setting: Hospice," 1975, paper submitted for partial fulfillment of psychology major, Florence and Henry Wald Papers, Yale University, New Haven, Connecticut.

For his thesis he drafted a blueprint Henry J. Wald, "A Hospice for Terminally Ill Patients," May 21, 1971, paper submitted for master's degree, Columbia University School of Architecture, Florence and Henry Wald Papers, Yale University, New Haven, Connecticut. Also, Joan Kron, "Designing a Better Place to Die," *The Hospice Concept: Introductory Essays and Bibliography,* ed. Roberta Halporn (Brooklyn: Highly Specialized Promotions, 1977).

reverence for life "Hospice Planning

Group Philosophy Statement," April 7, 1971, Edward J. Dobihal Jr. Papers, Yale University, New Haven, Connecticut. Also, Florence Wald and Sally S. Bailey, "Nurturing the Spiritual Component in Care for the Terminally Ill," *Caring Magazine* 9, no. 11 (November 1990).

Chapter 3: Cure Versus Care

Ninety-four percent of Americans live within an hour's drive Melissa D. A. Carlson, Elizabeth H. Bradley, Qingling Du, and R. Sean Morrison, "Geographic Access to Hospice in the United States," *Journal of Palliative Medicine* 13, no. 11 (November 2010): 1331–1338, accessed March 30, 2013, http://www.ncbi.nlm.nih.gov/pmc/articles/PMC3000898.

Two of them wound up in court David Wahlberg, "Madison Area Sees Increased Competition in Hospice Market," *Wisconsin State Journal,* September 4, 2011, accessed March 20, 2013, http://host.madison.com/news/local/health_med_fit/madison-area sees-increased-competition-in-hospice-market/article_3b22dd7e-d589-11e0-8903-001cc4c002e0.html.

When we tried to get our first hospice "Staying Home: A Guide to Hospices around the State," *Texas Monthly,* April

1981, accessed March 20, 2013, http://
books.google.com/books?id=ySwEAAAA
MBAJ&pg=PA162&lpg=PA162&dq=
texas+monthly+mary+mckenna+hospice
&source=bl&ots=wA0I2XxwEe&sig=Z-
KJVWrwNzJbKAZ-GL9LDfo77_g&hl=en
&sa=X&ei=gP1BUZGeO5Hl4APW-IHg
Dw&ved=0CDIQ6AEwAQ#v=onepage
&q=texas%20monthly%20mary%20mcken
na%20hospice&f=false.

**for-profit companies accounted for 60
percent of Medicare-certified hospice
providers** National Hospice and Palliative
Care Organization, *NHPCO Facts and Figures.*

pays the bills of 84 percent of patients
Ibid.

**The ideal of care driven solely by the
needs of patients collided with a system**
Paul. R. Torrens, ed., *Hospice Programs and
Public Policy* (Chicago: American Hospital
Publishing, Inc., 1985). Also, E.K. Abel,
"The Hospice Movement: Institutionalizing
Innovation," *International Journal of Health
Services* 16, no. 1 (1986): 71–85. Also, Joy
Buck, " 'I Am Willing to Take the Risk':
Politics, Policy, and the Translation of the
Hospice Ideal," *Journal of Clinical Nursing*
18, no. 19 (2009): 2700–2709.

What does hospice mean? Florence

363

Wald memo to Edward J. Dobihal Jr., "Reconstruction of the Meeting with Mr. Jarvis and Mr. Paterwic, May 14, 1971, 10:00 a.m.–11:40 a.m., Connecticut State Department of Health," May 18, 1971, Edward J. Dobihal Jr. Papers, Yale University, New Haven, Connecticut.

The part that was dropped all the time and **Under no circumstances will I ever send any child to hospice** Doris Howell interview, October 25, 1997, Hospice and Palliative Care Oral History Archive, School of Interdisciplinary Studies, University of Glasgow, Dumfries Campus.

We believed in the idea so much we weren't prepared Kerns, "A Study of the Creation of a Community Setting."

We are all so sorry that the thought of building Cicely Saunders to Florence Wald, December 15, 1973, Florence and Henry Wald Papers, Yale University, New Haven, Connecticut.

weeks, not months or years "Hospice Inc. Annual Report to National Institutes of Health," September 1, 1975, Edward J. Dobihal Papers, Yale University, New Haven, Connecticut. Also, Sylvia Lack, "New Haven (1974) — Characteristics of a Hospice Program of Care," *Death Education* 2, no. 1–2 (Spring/Summer 1978).

the tensions created by her Dennis Rezendes to Edward J. Dobihal, August 14, 1975, Florence and Henry Wald Papers, Yale University, New Haven, Connecticut.

I am somewhat distressed that the cost premise Bradford Gray, statement before the Subcommittee on Health, Committee on Ways and Means, House of Representatives, Hearing on Coverage of Hospice Under the Medicare Program, National Hospice Study Advisory Committee, March 25, 1982.

Chapter 4: House Calls

The medical student was surprised by her first hospice patient Paul R. Harnett and Timothy J. Moynihan, "But Doctor, What Have I Got to Lose . . . ?," *Journal of Clinical Oncology* 19, no. 13 (July 1, 2001). Also, Tracey A. Szirony, Patricia Sopko et al., "The Decision to Accept Hospice Services: A Qualitative Study," *Journal of Hospice and Palliative Nursing* 13, no. 5 (September/October 2011).

The largest study of its kind compared the survival rates Stephen R. Connor, Bruce Pyenson et al., "Comparing Hospice and Nonhospice Patient Survival Among Patients Who Die within a Three-Year Window," *Journal of Pain and Symptom Man-*

agement 33, no. 3 (March 2007).

Patients with congestive heart failure Ibid.

More than 11 percent National Hospice and Palliative Care Organization, *NHPCO Facts and Figures.* 2012 edition.

Chapter 5: A Fragile Family Peace

It is the most common lung cancer found in women Types and Staging of Lung Cancer, accessed March 30, 2013, *About.com,* http://lungcancer.about.com/od/typesoflungcancer/a/Lung-Adenocarcinoma.html.

It was set up much the way child development books offer tips Barbara Karnes, "Gone from My Sight," in Barbara Karnes, *End of Life Guidelines Series: A Compilation of Barbara Karnes Booklets* (Amazon Digital Services, Inc.: July 26, 2012), Kindle edition.

Chapter 6: Final Fast

Nobody would call the act suicide James L. Bernat, Bernard Gert, and R. Peter Mogielnicki, "Patient Refusal of Hydration and Nutrition: An Alternative to Physician-Assisted Suicide or Voluntary Active Euthanasia," *Archives of Internal Medicine* 153, no. 24 (December 27, 1993):

2723–2731.

The state Supreme Court ruled in 2009 Baxter v. Montana, 2009 MT 449 (December 31, 2009).

Law books do not say much about fasting Judith K. Schwarz, "Death by Voluntary Dehydration: Suicide or the Right to Refuse a Life-Prolonging Measure?" *Widener Law Review* 17 (2011): 351–361, accessed March 30, 2013, http://widener lawreview.org/files/2011/07/02-schwarz2 .pdf. Also, Judith Schwarz, "Exploring the Option of Voluntarily Stopping Eating and Drinking Within the Context of a Suffering Patient's Request for a Hastened Death," *Journal of Palliative Medicine* 10, no. 6 (December 2007): 1288–1297.

The only published study on the question Linda Ganzini, Elizabeth Goy et al., "Nurses' Experiences with Hospice Patients Who Refuse Food and Fluids to Hasten Death," *New England Journal of Medicine,* July 24, 2003, 349, 359–65, accessed March 30, 2013, http://www.nejm.org/doi/full/ 10.1056/NEJMsa035086#t=articleTop.

runs counter to the hospice philosophy Cicely Saunders, Templeton Prize Speech, May 1981, in Saunders, *Cicely Saunders.* Also, Cicely Saunders, "The

Management of Patients in the Terminal State," *Cancer* 6 (1960): 403–417.

85 to 95 percent of people in Oregon and Washington Courtney S. Campbell and Margaret A. Black, "Dignity, Death and Dilemmas: A Study of Washington Hospices and Physician-Assisted Death," *Journal of Pain and Symptom Management,* July 3, 2013, 270-274. Also, "Hospice Workers Struggle on Front Lines of Physician-Assisted Death Laws," *Oregon State University News and Research Communications,* July 22, 2013, accessed July 26, 2013, http:// oregonstate.edu/ua/ncs/archives/2013/jul/ hospice-workers-struggle-front-lines-physician-assisted-death-laws.

difference is not mere semantics Robert J. Sullivan, "Accepting Death without Artificial Nutrition or Hydration," *Journal of General Internal Medicine* 8, no. 4 (April 1993): 220-224.

Death by a thousand paper cuts "Debility Unspecified," *Hospice Doctor: Musings of a Specialist in End-of-Life Care* (blog), October 26, 2007, accessed March 30, 2013, http://hospicedoctor.blogspot.com/ 2007/10/debility-unspecified.html.

Betty would later reproduce the list Elizabeth S. Menkin, "Nourishment While

Fasting," *Journal of Palliative Medicine* 13, no. 10 (2010): 1288-1289.

Instead of drinking water, he drank from the wellsprings Ibid.

Chapter 7: Inside the Catch-22 of Hospice

Dying isn't hard. Getting paid by Medicare is Art Buchwald, *Too Soon to Say Goodbye* (New York: Random House, 2006).

Washington's Hottest Salon Sharon Waxman, "Washington's Hottest Salon Is a Deathbed," *New York Times,* Mar. 26, 2006.

having a swell time Buchwald, *Too Soon.*

Regina painted all summer, as an outlet for her grief and her anger Regina Holliday, "Dark Willow and '73 Cents' ", *Regina Holliday's Medical Advocacy Blog,* Sept. 25, 2009, accessed June 15, 2013, http://reginaholliday.blogspot.com.

***Buffy* was not afraid to talk about dying** Ibid.

Chapter 8: Up from the Abyss

they were having trouble sleeping, eating, concentrating National Institute on Aging, "Mourning the Death of a Spouse," National Institutes of Health, Age Page, January 2010, accessed March 14, 2013, http://www.nia.nih.gov/health/publication/

mourning-death-spouse.

Every year, nearly 1 million people in the United States lose their spouses Elizabeth J. Bergman and William E. Haley, "Depressive Symptoms, Social Network, and Bereavement Service Utilization and Preferences among Spouses of Former Hospice Patients," *Journal of Palliative Medicine* 12, no. 2 (2009).

grief is intensely personal Peter A. Beatty, "On the Death of a Spouse: Reflections of a Medical Oncologist," *Journal of Clinical Oncology* 22, no. 5 (March 1, 2004), 959-960, accessed March 30, 2013, http://jco.ascopubs.org/content/22/5/959.full.

Chapter 9: Turning Points

Research confirms the importance of laughter Bergman and Haley, "Depressive Symptoms." Also, Dale A. Lund, Rebecca Utz et al., "Humor, Laughter, and Happiness in the Daily Lives of Recently Bereaved Spouses," *Omega (Westport)* 58 no. 2 (2008–2009): 87–105, accessed March 14, 2013, http://www.ncbi.nim.nih.gov/pmc/articles/PMC2646184/.

how do you know that you really are climbing out of the abyss? Amanda L. Forte, Malinda Hill et al., "Bereavement Care Interventions: A Systematic Review,"

BMC Palliative Care 3 no. 3 (2004), accessed March 24, 2013, http://www.biomedcentral .com/1472-684X/3/3.

Medicare requires hospices Department of Health and Human Services, Centers for Medicare and Medicaid Services, "Medicare and Medicaid Programs: Hospice Conditions of Participation," *Federal Register* 73, no. 109 (June 5, 2008), accessed March 24, 2013, http://www.gpo.gov/ fdsys/pkg/FR-2008-06-05/pdf/08-1305.pdf.

The patient and family constitute the unit of care Sandol Stoddard, *The Hospice Movement: A Better Way of Caring for the Dying* (New York: Stein and Day, 1978). Also, Amanda Roberts and Sinead McGilloway, "The Nature and Use of Bereavement Support Services in a Hospice Setting," *Bereavement Care* 29, no. 1 (2010): 14-18.

Both facing loss and turning away are appropriate responses Colin Murray Parkes, "Grief: Lessons from the Past, Visions for the Future," *Death Studies* 26, no. 5 (June 2002): 367–385.

All this attention to survivors has sparked a nasty backlash Dale G. Larson and William T. Hoyt, "What Has Become of Grief Counseling? An Evaluation of the Empirical Foundations of the New Pessimism," *Professional Psychology: Research* *and Practice* 38, no. 4 (2007). Also, Sharon Begley, "Get Shrunk at Your Own Risk," *Newsweek,* June 18, 2007. Also, Allen Frances, "Don't Confuse Grief with Depression," *Huffington Post,* January 27, 2012.

the hospice industry paid 5,000 full-time employees in bereavement services Ruth Davis Konigsberg, *The Truth About Grief* (New York: Simon and Schuster, 2011).

critics to charge that DSM-5 Sarah Noel, "Good Grief: Why the DSM-V Is Wrong about Bereavement and Depression," *GoodTherapy.org* (blog), February 4, 2013, accessed March 30, 2013, http://www.good-therapy.org/blog/grief-bereavement-depression-dsm-v-0204134.

a temporary course of an antidepressant M. Katherine Shear, "Recognizing Complicated Grief and How to Help Patients through the Process," *Psychiatric Times,* October 21, 2011, accessed March 30, 2013, http://www.psychiatrictimes.com/mdd/content/article/10168/1974982.

For the vast majority Parkes, "Grief: Lessons from the Past, Visions for the Future," *Death Studies.*

Chapter 10: The Gift of Grace

Both patients pushed aside doubts Linda Emanuel, Katherine Bennett, and Virginia Richardson, "The Dying Role," *Journal of Palliative Medicine* 10, no. 1 (2007).

pain is not just a medical problem Cathy Siebold, *The Hospice Movement* (New York: Twayne Publishers, 1992).

The patient's first question Maggie Callanan and Patricia Kelley, *Final Gifts* (New York: Bantam, 2008).

Healing is distinguished from cure Christina Puchalski, Betty Ferrell et al., "Improving the Quality of Spiritual Care as a Dimension of Palliative Care: The Report of the Consensus Conference," *Journal of Palliative Medicine* 12, no. 10 (2009).

The volunteer has no agenda but to listen Hospice Foundation of America, "Volunteering and Hospice," accessed March 30, 2013, http://www.hospice foundation.org/volunteering.

Robert Butler, a pioneer of gerontology and a research psychiatrist, described a formal process for looking back on one's life Douglas Martin, "Robert Butler, Aging Expert, Is Dead at 83," *New York Times,* July 7, 2010. Also, Kenneth J. Doka and Amy S. Tucci, *Living With Grief: Spirituality and End-of-Life Care*

(Washington, D. C.: Hospice Foundation of America, 2011).

Being elderly was a life-cycle role Emanuel, Bennett, and Richardson, "The Dying Role."

Saunders's concept of total pain Andrew R. Barnosky, "Dignity Therapy: Final Words for Final Days," *Journal of the American Medical Association* 307, no. 23 (June 20, 2012): 2550.

Sometimes people want their families to know Lori Montross, Kathryn Winters, and Scott Irwin, "Dignity Therapy Implementation in a Community-Based Hospice Setting," *Journal of Palliative Medicine* 14, no. 6 (2011).

Making the Dignity Therapy recordings Susan McClement, Harvey Chochinov et al., "Dignity Therapy: Family Member Perspectives," *Journal of Palliative Medicine* 10, no. 5 (2007).

61 percent of people surveyed said a miracle could save a person Eric Widera, Kenneth Rosenfeld et al., "Approaching Patients and Family Members Who Hope for a Miracle," *Journal of Pain and Symptom Management* 42, no. 1 (2011): 119–25.

eighty-five fellowship programs in hospice and palliative medicine Fellowship Program Directory, American Academy of Hospice and Palliative Medicine, accessed March 30, 2013, http://www.aahpm.org/fellowship/default/fellowshipdirectory.html.

A thin veneer of physician arrogance Janne Fishman, letter to the editor, *New York Times,* March 15, 1996.

six of the nation's 126 medical schools required courses in end-of-life care Marilyn J. Field and Christine K. Cassel, eds., *Approaching Death: Improving Care at the End of Life,* Committee on Care at the End of Life, Institute of Medicine (Washington, D. C.: National Academy Press, 1997), accessed March 30, 2013, http://www.nap.edu/openbook.php?record_id=5801.

analysis of fifty major nursing education textbooks Betty R. Ferrell, Rose Virani, and Marcia Grant, "Analysis of Symptom Assessment and Management Content in Nursing Textbooks," *Journal of Palliative Medicine* 2, no. 2 (Summer 1999): 161–173.

Students at the University of Pittsburgh School of Medicine Wendy G. Anderson, Jillian E. Williams et al., "Exposure to Death Is Associated with Positive Attitudes and Higher Knowledge about

End-of-Life Care in Graduating Medical Students," *Journal of Palliative Medicine* 11, no. 9 (November 2008): 1227–1233, accessed March 30, 2013, http://www.ncbi.nlm.nih.gov/pmc/articles/PMC2941667/.

only 6 percent of interns (first-year doctors, training in hospitals) had experienced the death James L. Hallenbeck and Merlynn R. A. Bergen, "A Medical Resident Inpatient Hospice Rotation: Experiences with Dying and Subsequent Changes in Attitudes and Knowledge," *Journal of Palliative Medicine* 2, no. 2 (Summer 1999): 197–209.

one in five graduating medical students rated their instruction Association of American Medical Colleges, "2012 Medical School Graduation Questionnaire, All Schools Summary Report," accessed June 15, 2013, https://www.aamc.org/download/300448/data.

American Board of Internal Medicine made end-of-life instruction an education requirement Robert Wood Johnson Foundation, "End-of-Life Project Trains Medical Educators to Add Palliative Care Curriculum for Medical Residents," (October 2006), accessed March 30, 2013, http://pweb1.rwjf.org/reports/grr/046547.htm.

first exam to certify hospice and pal-

liative medicine as a subspecialty American Board of Internal Medicine, "Hospice and Palliative Medicine Policies," accessed March 30, 2013, http://www.abim.org/certification/policies/imss/hospice.aspx.

patients with terminal lung cancer, those who received palliative care Jennifer S. Temel, Joseph A. Greer et al., "Early Palliative Care for Patients with Metastatic Non-Small-Cell Lung Cancer," *New England Journal of Medicine* 363 (August 9, 2010): 733–742.

provisional recommendation that palliative care be incorporated into standard cancer oncology practice Thomas J. Smith, Sarah Temin, Erin R. Alesi et. al., "American Society of Clinical Oncology Provisional Clinical Opinion: The Integration of Palliative Care into Standard Oncology Care," *Journal of Clinical Oncology* 30, no. 8 (March 10, 2012): 880–887.

stories about patients in the ICU Lauren Van Scoy, *Last Wish: Stories to Inspire a Peaceful Passing* (Austin: Transmedia Books, 2012).

850,000 licensed physicians Aaron Young, Humayun J. Chaudry et al., "A Census of Actively Licensed Physicians in the United States, 2010." *Journal of Medical Regulation* 96, no. 4 (2010): 10–20, ac-

cessed July 10, 2013, http://www.national
ahec.org/pdfs/FSMBPhysicianCensus.pdf.

hope is connected to the future Sher-
win B. Nuland, "The Doctor's Role in
Death," in *Facing Death: Where Culture,
Religion, and Medicine Meet,* eds. Howard
Spiro, Mary G. McCrea Curnen, and Lee
Palmer Wandel, (New Haven: Yale Univer-
sity Press, 1998).

Chapter 12: Dying for Dollars
**sleep in the White House Lincoln Bed-
room** "The Lincoln Bedroom Guest List,"
February 25, 1997, *AllPolitics,* accessed
March 20, 2013, http://edition.cnn.com/
ALLPOLITICS/1997/02/25/clinton.money/
list.html.

**11,000 employees in fifty-one pro-
grams** "Chemed Corporation Results as of
December 2012," presentation at Barclay's
Healthcare Conference, March 13, 2013,
accessed March 30, 2013, http://ir .chemed
.com/phoenix.zhtml?p=irol-eventDetails&
c=72704&eventID=4926033.

**Chemed president and CEO, earned
$6.4 million** Chemed Corporation, *2011
Annual Report,* http://phx.corporate-ir.net/
External.File?item=UGFyZW50SUQ9MT
M0MDA1fENoaWxkSUQ9LTF8VHlwZT0
z&t=1. Also, Chemed Corporation, 2012

Proxy Statement, accessed March 30, 2013, http://phx.corporate-ir.net/External.File?item=UGFyZW50SUQ9NDYxMzI0fEN oaWxkSUQ9NDg5NjJAfFR5cGU9MQ= =&t=1.

60 percent of Medicare-certified hospice providers were for-profit companies National Hospice and Palliative Care Organization, *NHPCO Facts and Figures.*

Gentiva operated hospice programs in 165 locations across thirty states Gentiva Health Services, SEC10-K Annual Report for 2012, accessed March. 30, 2013 http://investors.gentiva.com/common/ download/download.cfm?companyid= GTIV&fileid=649439&filekey=c19b772a-98ce-4d20-8d5f-3b194bd2e597&filename= Gentiva_2012_Annual_Report.pdf.

Hospice deal volume continues to roll Scott Becker, Krist Werling, and Holly Carnell, "Private Equity Investing in Health Care — 13 Hot and 4 Cold Areas," *Becker's Hospital Review,* August 16, 2011, accessed March 30, 2013, http://www.beckershospital review.com/hospital-management-adminis tration/private-equityinvesting-in-health care-13-hot-and-4-cold-areas.html.

mission to generate attractive investment returns "Our Mission," *Sentinel Capital Partners,* accessed July 10, 2013,

http://sentinelpartners.com/secondary.asp?
pageID=3.

ongoing strategy of investing in companies with demonstrated earnings potential Steven Mufson, "Washington Post Co. Buys Hospice Firm Celtic Healthcare," *Washington Post,* October. 1, 2012, accessed July 10, 2013, http://articles.washingtonpost.com/2012-10-01/business/35500763_1_hospice-homecare-foray-into-healthcare.

A blistering investigation by Bloomberg reporter Peter Waldman, "Aunt Midge Not Dying in Hospice Reveals $14B Market," *Bloomberg,* December 5, 2011, accessed March 30, 2013, http://www.bloomberg.com/news/2011-12-06/hospice-care-revealed-as-14-billion-u-s-market.html. Also, Peter Waldman, "Preparing Americans for Death Lets Hospices Neglect End of Life," *Bloomberg,* July 22, 2011, http://www.bloomberg.com/news/2011-07-22/preparing-americans-for-death-lets-for-profit-hospices-neglect-end-of-life.html. Also, Peter Waldman, "Hospices Dump Patients, Escape Millions Owed," *Bloomberg,* February 2, 2012, http://www.bloomberg.com/news/2012-02-03/hospices-dump-patients-while-escaping-multimillion-dollar-taxpayer-refunds.html.

a longtime hospice nurse, Nancy Costea, published a powerful essay Nancy Costea, "Are You My Nurse? Life and Death in the Hospice Fast Lane," *Nursing Forum* 46, no. 4 (October–December 2011): 251–255.

for-profits have proportionally fewer high-end professionals Emily J. Cherlin, Melissa D. A. Carlson et al., "Interdisciplinary Staffing Patterns: Do For-Profit and Nonprofit Hospices Differ?" *Journal of Palliative Medicine* 13, no. 4 (2010): 389–94.

A study of 1,036 hospice agencies Melissa W. Wachterman, Edward R. Marcantonio et al., "Association of Profit Status and Diagnosis with Hospice Care," *Journal of the American Medical Association* 305, no. 5 (February 2, 2011): 472–479, accessed March 30, 2013, http://www.ncbi.nlm.nih.gov/pmc/articles/PMC3142476/.

palliative radiation can run about $7,500 Gregory Hess, Arie Barlev et al., "Cost of Palliative Radiation to the Bone for Patients with Bone Metastases Secondary to Breast or Prostate Cancer," *Radiation Oncology* 7, no. 168 (2012), accessed March 30, 2013, http://www.ro-journal.com/content/7/1/168.

A unit of blood ranges from $500 to

$1,200 Aryeh Shander, Axel Hofmann et al., "Activity-Based Costs of Blood Transfusions in Surgical Patients at Four Hospitals," *Transfusion* 50, no. 4 (April 2010): 753–765, accessed March 30, 2013, http://onlinelibrary.wiley.com/doi/10.1111/j.15372995.2009.02518.x/full.

Carol and Joe sued VITAS Hargett v. Vitas Healthcare Corp., No. RG10547255 (Cal. Super. Ct., filed on November 18, 2010).

$45.48 a day per patient for routine home care Mary Cummings, "Current Status of Hospice Financing," in *Hospice Programs and Public Policy,* ed. Paul R. Torrens (Chicago: American Hospital Publishing, Inc., 1985).

fewer than 10 percent applied Ibid.

A 1993 investigation by the *Miami New Times* Jim DeFede, "Death and Profits," *Miami New Times,* June 16, 1993, accessed March 30, 2013, http://www.miaminewtimes.com/1993-06-16/news/death-and-profits/.

Investors like the large under-serviced market Steve Gelsi, "Odyssey Makes IPO Journey: CEO Floated IPO on Strong Balance Sheet," November 28, 2001, *CBS MarketWatch,* accessed March 30, 2013, http://www.marketwatch.com/story/odysseyhealth

care-ceo-says-profits-prompted-ipo.

Medicare spending for hospice has shot up Medicare Payment Advisory Commission, *Report to the Congress: Medicare Payment Policy,* accessed March 30, 2013, http://www.medpac.gov/chapters/Mar12_Ch11.pdf.

hospice use by Alzheimer's and dementia patients Centers for Medicare and Medicaid Services, *Hospice Data 1998–2008,* http://www.cms.gov/Medicare/Medicare-Fee-for-Service-Payment/Hospice/Downloads/Hospice_Data_1998-2008.zip.

pay $1.3 million to settle charges that it had falsely billed Medicare Department of Justice, Office of Public Affairs, "South Carolina-Based Harmony Care Hospice, Inc., and CEO/Owner Daniel J. Burton to Pay U.S. $1.286 Million to Resolve False Claims Act Allegations," November 20, 2012, accessed March 30, 2013, http://www.justice.gov/opa/pr/2012/November/12-civ-1401.html.

settled similar charges, for $6.1 million Department of Justice, Office of Public Affairs, "Hospice Care of Kansas and Texas-Based Parent Company to Pay $6.1 Million to Resolve Allegations of False Claims," June 21, 2012, accessed March 30, 2013, http://www.justice.gov/opa/pr/2012/June/12-

civ-768.html.

Odyssey did too, in March 2012, for $25 million Gentiva Health Services, SEC Form 8-K, February 21, 2012, accessed March 30, 2013, http://biz.yahoo.com/e/120221/gtiv8-k.html.

an unmitigated tragedy "End of an Era," *Hospice Doctor: Musings of a Specialist in End-of-Life Care* (blog), March 17, 2013, accessed July 10, 2013, http://hospicedoctor.blogspot.com/2013_03_01_archive.html.

Scripps CEO Chris Van Gorder publicly pledged a commitment Kathleen Pacurar and Chris Van Gorder, "Difficult Transitions: Scripps Can Carry on Legacy of San Diego Hospice," *San Diego Union-Tribune,* February 23, 2013, accessed March 30, 2013, http://www.utsandiego.com/news/2013/feb/23/scripps-sandiego-hospice-care/?page=2.

demonstration projects around the country to test a concept called "concurrent care" The Patient Protection and Affordable Care Act, Pub. L. No. 111-148, § 3140 (2010), accessed March 30, 2013, http://www.gpo.gov/fdsys/pkg/PLAW-111publ148/html/PLAW-111publ148.htm.

Hospice use more than doubled Claire M. Spettell, Wayne Rawlins et al., "A Comprehensive Case Management Program to Improve Palliative Care," *Journal of Palliative Medicine* 12, no. 9 (2009): 827–832.

Chapter 13: Cultural Revolutions
more than 80 percent of hospice patients are white Hospice Foundation of America, "Addressing Cultural Diversity in Hospice," accessed March 30, 2013, www .hospicefoundation.org/uploads/hic_fs_ diversity.pdf.

much more likely to have heard about hospice Elizabeth K. Vig, Helene Starks et al., "Why Don't Patients Enroll in Hospice? Can We Do Anything About It?" *Journal of General Internal Medicine* 25, no. 10 (October 2010): 1009–1019, accessed March 14, 2013, http://www.ncbi.nlm.nih.gov/pmc/ articles/PMC2955487/. Also, Amber E. Barnato, Denise L. Anthony et al., "Racial and Ethnic Differences in Preferences for End-of-Life Treatment," *Journal of General Internal Medicine* 24, no. 6 (June 2009): 695–701, accessed March 14, 2013, http:// www.ncbi.nlm.nih.gov/pmc/articles/PMC 2686762/. Also, Marjorie Kagawa-Singer and Leslie J. Blackhall, "Negotiating Cross-Cultural Issues at the End of Life: 'You Got to Go Where He Lives,' " *Journal of the American Medical Association* 286, no. 23 (December 19, 2001).

I thought it was a place worse than a hospital Vig, Starks et al., "Why Don't Patients Enroll in Hospice?"

Death and dying are topics that many Latinos may not be willing Silvia Austerlic, "Cultural Humility and Compassionate Presence at the End of Life," Santa Clara University Markkula Center for Applied Ethics, accessed June 27, 2013, http://www.scu.edu/ethics/practicing/focusareas/medical/culturally-competent-care/chronic-to-critical-austerlic.html.

Chinese Americans are five times more likely than Caucasians to die with feeding tubes Paul Stokes and Sandy Chen Stokes, "Doing Everything We Can," Hospice Foundation of America newsletter, *Journeys,* Chinese Issue, 2009.

the nineteenth-century Opium Wars Philip V. Allingham, "England and China: The Opium Wars," *The Victorian Web: Literature, History, and Culture in the Age of Victoria,* accessed March 30, 2013, http://www.victorianweb.org/history/empire/opiumwars/opiumwars1.html. Also, Karl E. Mayer, "The Opium Wars' Secret History," *New York Times,* June 28, 1997.

families do not speak about death with the loved one who is dying "Loving Life: Understanding Hospice Care," Chinese

American Coalition for Compassionate Care, www.caccc-usa.org, DVD.

hospice use by African Americans National Hospice and Palliative Care Organization, *NHPCO Facts and Figures.*

religious beliefs about God's will Pew Research, "A Religious Portrait of African-Americans," last updated January 30, 2009, http://www.pewforum.org/A-Religious-Portrait-of-African-Americans.aspx.

Hospice staff need to know about *curanderismo* Sylvia Austerlic, "Grief and Loss in the Latino Family," summary from *Mensajeros de Confianza,* Hospice of Santa Cruz County, May 30, 2008.

The worst thing about hospice care? Barbara Kreling, Claire Selsky et al., " 'The Worst Thing About Hospice Is That They Talk about Death': Contrasting Hospice Decisions and Experience Among Immigrant Central and South American Latinos with U.S.-Born White, Non-Latino Caregivers," *Palliative Medicine* 24, no. 4 (2010): 427–434.

First-generation Latino immigrants Austerlic, "Grief and Loss."

a trial period of music therapy Elizabeth Joy Gifford, "The Experience of African American Hospice Patient/Family with Board-Certified Music Therapy as a Component of their Plan of Care" (doctor of nursing practice thesis, University of San Francisco, 2009), 14.

Chapter 14: Not If, But When

"the disconnect" between the needs of the health care system and those of patients Rebecca L. Sudore and Terri R. Fried, "Redefining the 'Planning' in Advance Care Planning: Preparing for End-of-Life Decision Making," *Annals of Internal Medicine* 153, no. 4 (August 17, 2010): 256–261.

She wrote about the incident Rebecca L. Sudore, "Can We Agree to Disagree?" *Journal of the American Medical Association* 302, no. 15 (October 21, 2009): 1629–1630.

She told me that she loved my grandfather Ibid.

because she would have to live with her decision Ibid.

In a study of patients with advanced cancer Angelo E. Volandes, Michael K. Paasche-Orlow et al., "Randomized Controlled Trial of a Video Decision Support Tool for Cardiopulmonary Resuscitation Decision-Making in Advanced Cancer," *Journal of Clinical Oncology* 31, no. 3 (January 2013): 380–386.

Reflections

We're all patients Tara Parker Pope, "We're All Patients," *New York Times,* Feb. 19, 2013.

I cry a lot because I miss people. . . . They die and I can't stop them NPR, "Fresh Air Remembers Author Maurice Sendak," last updated May 8, 2012, http://www.npr.org/2012/05/08/152248901/fresh-air-remembersauthormaurice-sendak.

Stephen Kiernan says Michael Bernhagen and Terry Kaldhusdal, *Consider the Conversation: A Documentary on a Taboo Subject* (2011), DVD.

INDEX

Medicare (*Cont.*)
  hospice benefit 98, 99, 175, 303
  regulations 79, 97, 103
  services 29, 30, 79, 82, 98, 99, 175,
      189–90, 212, 256, 273, 281, 284–85,
      291, 303
  fraud investigations 278, 292, 297, 298
medicine, palliative (*see* palliative
      medicine)
Meek, Carrie 94
Miami Dade College 94
Miami New Times 292
Memorial Sloan-Kettering Cancer Center
      60
Menkin, Elizabeth 102, 144, 248, 250,
      255, 261–70, 322, 323–24
mergers 274
miracles, belief in 31, 102, 244
Montross, Lori 237, 242
morphine 45, 146, 158, 286, 310
Mother Mary Alphonsa 62
Mount Holyoke College 69
Mukherjee, Siddhartha 38
National Cancer Institute 88
National Hospice Organization 30
National Steinbeck Center 130
New York Cancer Hospital 60
New York City Lunatic Asylum 59
Nguyen, Thuy 248, 249–50, 271
Nuland, Sherwin 271

nurses/nursing 30, 37, 39, 45, 47, 51–55,
        58, 60, 63–75, 78–81, 84–89, 92, 95,
        97–103, 113, 114, 120, 122, 129, 132,
        137, 140, 147–51, 158, 172–81, 189,
        230, 232, 239, 246, 252, 264, 266,
        272, 277–82, 289, 292, 296, 298, 302,
        318, 337, 343
Nursing Forum 278
nursing homes 30, 77–84, 94, 103, 109,
        148, 160, 236, 248, 250, 261, 262,
        289, 295, 297, 330
Oates, Joyce Carol 198
Obama, Barack 98, 144, 178
Odyssey HealthCare 278, 281, 293–94, 296
Office of Inspector General, Department of
        Health and Human Services 297
On Death and Dying 70, 217
On Grief and Grieving 217
Opium Wars 310
O'Toole, Timothy S. 275
Our Lady's Hospice 49
Our Lady Star of the Sea Church 316
pain
  control of 30, 42, 45, 66, 81, 165, 172,
        284
  denial of 217
  of dying person 28, 33, 40, 60, 71, 110,
        139, 142, 143, 149, 158, 166, 170–71,
        172, 176, 187, 189, 191, 197, 226–29,
        245, 252, 257, 264, 285

403

ABOUT THE AUTHORS

Fran Smith is a writer, editor, writing coach, and communications consultant. Her work has appeared in *O, The Oprah Magazine; Redbook; Salon; Good Housekeeping; Prevention; Health;* the *Los Angeles Times; USA Today;* and dozens of other publications and websites. She has won many awards for medical reporting, health care investigations, and feature writing, and shared in a Pulitzer Prize as a reporter at the *San Jose Mercury News.* Fran coauthored the first reporters' guidebook published by the Association of Health Care Journalists, and she is a frequent speaker on the power of storytelling, health care writing, and effective communications. She lives in New York with her husband and daughter.

Sheila Himmel is a *Psychology Today* blogger and coauthor of *Hungry: A Mother and Daughter Fight Anorexia* (Penguin,

2009). She is a contributor to *Restoring Our Bodies, Reclaiming Our Lives* (April 2011). Sheila writes for publications ranging from the *New York Times* to *Eating Well* to *IEEE Spectrum: The Magazine of Technology Insiders.* Her work has appeared in *USA Today,* the *Washington Post,* the *Robb Report, M Magazine* and the online magazine *Obit.* As restaurant critic of the *San Jose Mercury News,* Sheila won a James Beard Award for feature writing. She lives in the San Francisco Bay Area.

Fran and Sheila write the *Psychology Today* blog, "Changing the Way We Die." Visit them and learn the latest at www.changing thewaywedie.com.